Optimum Health the Paleo Way

Boost Energy Levels, Eliminate Sugar Cravings,
Reduce Processed Foods, Find Your Ideal Weight,
Develop an Eating Plan That Works for You, Sleep
Well & Feel Great!
Claire Yates BHSc

D1561151

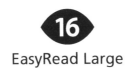

EasyRead Large

Copyright Page from the Original Book

First published 2013
Exisle Publishing Pty Ltd
'Moonrising', Narone Creek Road, Wollombi, NSW 2325, Australia
P.O. Box 60–490, Titirangi, Auckland 0642, New Zealand
www.exislepublishing.com

Copyright © 2013 in text: Claire Yates
Copyright © 2013 in photographs: Claire Yates
Claire Yates asserts the moral right to be identified as the author
of this work.

All rights reserved. Except for short extracts for the purpose of review,
no part of this book may be reproduced, stored in a retrieval system or
transmitted in any form or by any means, whether electronic, mechanical,
photocopying, recording or otherwise, without prior written permission
from the publisher.

National Library of Australia Cataloguing-in-Publication Data:

    Yates, Claire, author.

    Optimum health the Paleo way / Claire Yates BHSc.

    ISBN 978 1 921966 26 2 (pbk)

    Includes bibliographical references and index.

    High-protein diet.

    Prehistoric peoples—Nutrition.

    613.25

Design and typesetting by Tracey Gibbs
Illustrations by Country Charm Sketch Font
Typeset in Chaparral

EPub Edition © 2013 ISBN: 9781775591153

Disclaimer

While this book is intended as a general information resource and all care
has been taken in compiling the contents, this book does not take account
of individual circumstances and is not a substitute for medical advice.

Always consult a qualified practitioner or therapist. Neither the author nor
the publisher and their distributors can be held responsible for any loss,
claim or action that may arise from reliance on the information contained in
this book.

TABLE OF CONTENTS

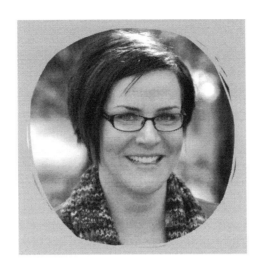

Claire Yates is a Nutritional Medicine Practitioner, holding a Bachelor of Health science, who is passionate about paleo nutrition, health and having fun! a self-confessed lover of good food and good coffee, Claire believes that living your best life and eating healthy food should not be boring. You can feel great from the inside out and still enjoy some of the tastiest food of your life! Through sharing her knowledge and 'walking the walk', Claire inspires people to enjoy nutritious, delectable food and live a fulfilling, healthy life. a former lecturer in nutritional medicine, Claire currently runs her own private practice, Indi Nature. For more information on Claire and her work, visit w ww.indinature.com

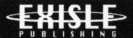 **e-newsletter**

If you love books as much as we do, why not subscribe
to our weekly e-newsletter?

As a subscriber, you'll receive special offers and discounts,
be the first to hear of our exciting upcoming titles, and
be kept up to date with book tours and author events.
You will also receive unique opportunities exclusive
to subscribers – and much more!

To subscribe in Australia or from any other
country except New Zealand, visit
www.exislepublishing.com.au/newsletter-sign-up

For New Zealand, visit
www.exislepublishing.co.nz/newsletter-subscribe

To my husband Paul—thank you for believing in, supporting and adventuring through life with me.

Introduction

I'm a nutritionist, so I guess that must mean that I am blessed with gorgeous skin and a perfect body, I never get stressed and eat only organic, green food ALL the time, right?

That statement couldn't be further from the truth, except the part about me being a nutritionist—I have the degree on the wall to prove that one!

Over the years, while practising as a nutritionist, I have learnt many things about myself, but I think one of the most important things has been that every person's nutritional needs are individual. So often we read about how something is good for us or something is not good, or we should be eating 'X' amount of something if we want to be healthy or only a small portion of 'Y' if we want to lose weight. But, you know what? WE ARE ALL INDIVIDUAL! Goji berries might be the best super food in the world, but it does not mean they are right for everyone. Low-carb eating may have worked for some people, but that doesn't mean it is right for you.

Food is fundamental to our life—we all need to eat! What you may not know, however, is that how much of what you eat not only affects your weight, but also your health, happiness and outlook on life. But food is just one part of the puzzle; there are many other factors just as important to good health.

Through this book I want to share with you the 'bigger picture' relating to our health—what has happened to it, how our food system has changed, and how things like stress play a crucial role in our health. Hormones, gut bugs, inflammation, sleep and nature are all very important parts of the health puzzle, so it is important to get a better understanding of how they all connect to our wellbeing.

Adopting a Paleo template is essentially about eating fewer processed whole foods that do not cause you any ill effects (for example, possibly excluding foods such as some grains, dairy and legumes, as these can upset many). Sounds easy enough, but it can be a bit overwhelming in the beginning. I have included a great 28-day Reset protocol to help you start eating the Paleo way—and I give you guidance and tips on how to stick to the template, while still allowing you to make individualised choices to suit you.

I will help you with food choices, stocking your pantry and deciding what to eat for the first few weeks to get you started. I even have over 100 yummy recipes for you to try! You don't have to worry about restrictive eating; these recipes are easy to make, taste great and are packed full of nutrients.

While you are reading this book, I would like you to take the information given and test things out for yourself, because ultimately, no one knows your body better than you. You may be feeling unwell, lethargic or just out-of-sorts because you simply have forgotten how to listen to your body. We are all guilty of that! To start to feel good again, all you need to do is allow your body time to heal after getting off the junk food you have been eating. Begin treating your body as a whole by evaluating your lifestyle and eating habits and learn to recognise what is right for your body and what is not. Treat your body with love, nourish it with proper *real food* and it will look after you in return. Turn off the TV, tune in to your loved ones, feel the dirt on your feet, eat wholesome food and start to feel alive. There is no better way of looking after your health and wellbeing than investing time in *you.* No one else can do that for you and I'm sorry, no magic pill will do it either!

Now, there are certain parts of the book I would like to draw your attention to, especially if you are a bit of a closet nerd and like to geek out a bit! Several question-and-answer sections are featured, which provide further in-depth information relating to the chapter topic and particular functional pathology testing that may be considered. These questions are answered by Warren Maginn, a savvy dude when it comes to nutritional medicine but also, technically, a functional clinical nutritionist and educator. He is the National Technical Educator for Research Nutrition, where he supports and educates naturopathic and medical practitioners in the use of functional pathology testing and he also lectures in Nutritional Medicine at the Endeavour College of Natural Medicine. I am very grateful to Warren for giving his time and expertise to this book.

So, how did I get here?

Growing up, I always loved food. I remember always wanting to bake and make different things in the kitchen. I grew up mainly a vegetarian, but I remember eating chicken and fish on the odd occasion. Many of our evening meals were made up of lots of raw vegetables from the garden and, going by typical Western diets, we ate fairly well. What I did eat a lot of, however, was sweets, baked goodies and other high-GI carbohydrates, like hot chips.

I was always a chubby kid and didn't really like participating in sports. Looking back on it now, I think it had to do with my height, or rather, my insecurity about my height. From memory, I think I was at the height I am today (183cm/6ft) when I was around thirteen or fourteen years old, and for a girl, that's tough to get used to. I always felt like everyone was looking at me, and that people wanted me to play what I would term 'tall people sports', such as netball and basketball. I also felt that people expected me to be a lot older because of my height and therefore treated me that way—like I was an adult.

...I was looking great, and I was encouraged to keep up the good work, but somewhere along the way something else happened. In my brain

> something changed, this 'weight thing' began to control *me.*

About the age of fourteen something happened. I didn't want to be looked at anymore; I just wanted to blend in. I wanted to be treated like the insecure, young teenage girl I was, not this grown woman who could apparently handle the world. This meant that I needed to take control of something, which at the time, happened to be my weight.

At first it was all good. I started a diet and exercise regime and began to lose weight. People congratulated me, I was looking great, and I was encouraged to keep up the good work, but somewhere along the way something else happened. In my brain something changed; this 'weight thing' began to control *me.* I felt like it was the one constant in my life over which I had control. When everything else around me was chaos, I could still control my weight and what I put in my mouth. Looking back now and after many years of therapy, I also know that because I lost too much weight and looked frail, people treated me how I felt—like a little girl who needed help, not some big tough Amazonian woman who could conquer the world.

I survived on little more than coffee, lettuce leaves, laxatives and exercise, and drove my family to despair. I ended up in treatment, but never really followed through, as once I started to gain weight I convinced everyone I was all right. The thing about *those years* was that I could tell you every calorie in every food, but nothing else. Not what vitamins or minerals were in it, how it could nourish your body or how it could benefit your health. I was only interested in 'calories in' and 'calories out'.

Fast-forward through my early adulthood and a pattern emerged of me just replacing my food control/addiction with another addiction, whether if be coffee, alcohol or even work. I always had something else in my life I needed to control. During those years, however, I still had emotional issues with food and could not resist the lure of chocolate or sweet foods and would continue to punish myself after not having the willpower to resist them.

> When I adopted this [paleo] template for myself, my weight normalised, I slept better (much better!), I didn't get headaches anymore, and I wasn't falling asleep at 2p.m. every afternoon!

So this brings me to my studies in nutrition. What better way to reform a person with an eating disorder and food addiction than to teach them all about nutrition? It combined all the things I loved—food, health and the need to nurture other people.

Studying nutrition was amazing and taught me how complex our bodies are and how important nutrients are for every facet of the body, from hormone production to the beating of our hearts. It taught me that calories don't really matter—food as medicine matters. I also found out about my love for biochemistry!

What studying nutrition did not teach me, however, was how to control my sugar cravings. I began to find again and again that the more stressed I felt, the more I reached for my coffee and a chocolate—typical life of a student, hey? I told myself, 'I will just lose this weight *after* I finish my degree.'

In my first year out of university, however, things did not change. I was sleepy at 2p.m., always wanted coffee and could NOT walk past the chocolate aisle in a supermarket without having a sneaky treat and then hating myself for it afterwards. How could I be a practising nutritionist, telling my clients to 'eat this and don't eat that' when as soon as I have them out the door I am reaching for my coffee and a muffin?

My weight was slowly creeping up despite my daily running and I was beginning to get very depressed and frustrated. My sleep was terrible and I could not control my eating. I was a failure at the very thing I was meant to be teaching people—how to eat for good health and wellbeing, and how to use food as medicine.

Enter Paleo. I don't know how I stumbled across this one little word, but it had a big impact on me. I began researching and researching. The science made sense, but why was I not taught this at university? Wholegrains are your friends, right?

I decided to do a little experiment, with me as the guinea pig. I cleaned out my kitchen pantry, ditched the foods that were problematic for me and began to eat *real food.* The result was that I corrected the hormonal imbalances I had been suffering from ever since my eating disorder, which I had never previously addressed. I also looked at the Paleo template a little differently through naturopathic eyes—meaning, that I also knew the importance of individuality when looking at dietary plans. I realised that treating the whole person was essential and lifestyle choices really, really matter!

When I adopted this template for myself, my weight normalised, I slept better (much better!), I didn't get headaches anymore, and I wasn't falling asleep at 2p.m. every afternoon! I also realised that I'm not missing out on anything. I am a real foodie and I am eating the most nourishing food I have ever eaten in my life and it tastes good! It all came down to understanding that this is not a diet, but a lifestyle choice. This is why I want to inspire you to find your true, healthy, individual nature through this book.

part 1

The Paleo Template

CHAPTER 1

Our health is the sum of many small parts

What is wrong with our health today? Is fructose to blame? Is sugar to blame? Is processed food to blame? Or is fat to blame? The answer is none of the above. You see, nothing to do with our health, food or nutrition is ever that black and white. We need to stop trying to point the finger at one single thing, because it just does not work that way. Our health is the sum of many small parts. Nobody develops obesity, arthritis or leaky-gut syndrome overnight. These conditions happen gradually and are an end-product of the choices an individual has made regarding their food intake and lifestyle.

So, what are some of the things that are negatively impacting our health today?

- Over-processed foods

2

- Inactive lifestyles

- Monumental increases in stress

- City living

- Disconnection from the community

- Disconnection from nature

- Sleep deprivation

- Disconnection from our food and farming

- Wanting a quick and easy solution (pill fix) to current health issues

- Too much technology

- A 24-hour lifestyle.

In the Western world, we have the highest rates of obesity, allergies, disease and ill health that we have ever seen. Something has to give and it is obvious that the current 'answers' to looking after our 'health' are not working. Who wants to keep popping pills and going on yo-yo diets in order to feel healthy? Being on countless medications and slimming shakes should not be the norm. Our quality of life seems to be slipping further and further towards ill health.

When we look at health, all aspects of our life need to be considered. It is not just about what food you put in your mouth. If you want to be the healthiest version of 'you' and have 'optimum health', you need to address all the areas in your life.

The World Health Organization defines health as:

> *...a state of complete physical, mental and social well-being and not merely the absence of disease or infirmity.*

This means we have a large percentage of the population out there walking around stressed, sick and unhealthy. Just because you do not have a disease does not mean you are healthy. And it is not just a single one of those elements I mentioned above that is doing the most damage to our health. It is a cumulative effect of all of them. And I am sure you could also add more elements to this list.

When we look at health, all aspects of our life need to be considered. It is not just about what food you put in your mouth. If you want to be the healthiest version of 'you' and have 'optimum health', you need to address all the areas in your life.

So, how do you obtain good health?

You start to turn the tables by incorporating small changes into your life that positively impact your health.

As author Alvin Toffler writes, *You've got to think about big things while you're doing small things, so that all the small things go in the right direction.*

In order to do this you first need to understand and recognise how your food choices and your lifestyle affect your health. You then need to be prepared to make some changes (possibly difficult ones to begin with) in order to better your health. You also need to understand that some of these changes may seem small and insignificant but, trust me, they will improve your health.

It's important that you take responsibility for your health and value it. Don't just expect it to take care of itself or try to fix it only after it has broken (although if it is already broken, you're in the right place to fix it), and certainly don't put your health in the hands of others to look after. A good holistic GP, nutritionist or naturopath can offer you knowledge and guidance, and give you the tools to get started on the road to good health but, ultimately, the control still lies with you. It is your job to make the changes and figure out what is right for you, and a good practitioner will encourage this process. Everyone can make *some* changes to better their health, including me! It's always a work in progress. It's about continually reviewing this process and seeing where you are at, as an individual. *You* are responsible for *your* health, so start making some changes now so you are on track to adding up your 'sum of small parts' to *good health.*

CHAPTER 2

Is that food or a bunch of chemicals?

Adopting a Paleo eating plan is not just about identifying what 'is' or 'is not' Paleo. It is also about acknowledging that what we eat plays a very important part in our health and that a lot of 'health foods' out there are not necessarily good for our health. An example is the amount of gluten-free products now available in supermarkets. Just because it is gluten free doesn't mean it is good for you. Most of that stuff is still over processed and full of sugar, hydrogenated fats, preservatives and additives.

What we call food has changed a lot over the past 50 years. You only need to take a walk through a supermarket and see what goes in the trolley of a family for their average weekly shop. How much of the *food* in their trolley would go mouldy or off in a few days? Not much! The majority of it would most likely have expiry dates of six months or longer. I'm sorry, but *real food* does not last! It decomposes and goes mouldy—a sign that something may be worthy of eating. Living, natural foods contain enzymes and it is these enzymes that cause the breakdown of foods through oxidation, browning and ripening. Packaged foods are filled with preservatives and additives to prevent spoilage and it is these guys you want to avoid in your food. I cover more about additives and preservatives in the next chapter.

> *Real food* does not last! It decomposes and goes mouldy—a sign that something may be worthy of eating.

So, what is food?

Now this is one of the few times you should believe Wikipedia! If you type in 'define food' you get this from the almighty oracle:

> *Food is any substance consumed to provide nutritional support for the body. It is usually of plant or animal origin, and contains essential nutrients, such as carbohydrates, fats, proteins, vitamins, or minerals. The substance is ingested by an organism and assimilated by the organism's cells in an effort to produce energy, maintain life, or stimulate growth.*
>
> *Historically, people secured food through two methods: hunting and gathering, and agriculture. Today, most of the food energy consumed by the world population is supplied by the food industry.*

Hmm ... so today we get most of our 'food' from the food industry? And it is that 'food' that is loading you up with empty, nutrient-LACKING calories (energy)! At a guess, I would hedge my bets that this is where most of our current 'lifestyle' health issues begin too. We are not eating real food anymore. We are eating processed 'food-like substances' made and packaged by the 'food industry' and we are paying the price. So, what is wrong with having a diet primarily based on these 'food-like substances'? I am going to have to pick a few key points to explain this, as I could write an entire book about this subject alone!

Inflammation and omega-6 fatty acids

I want to flag something here: inflammation. We have a whole chapter coming up on this, but for now just know that a lot of the health conditions prevalent in society today stem from chronic inflammation. You see, when your body is inflamed, it is like having a constant low-grade infection, like your body is always trying to fight off something. So it makes sense that if you are always in this state, you are more susceptible to other immune-related conditions, such as asthma or allergies. You know what you feel like if you've had a long hard day at work and then a lousy night's sleep? Do you perform well the next day? Of course not! Well, imagine that is your immune system and you never give it a day off. It is tired and overworked, which equals you being more susceptible to illness—makes sense?

So, now that we understand that, where does a lot of this inflammation come from? Excess omega-6!

Omega-3 and omega-6 are fatty acids, meaning they have a head (carboxylic acid) and a tail of various lengths made up of carbon links—they are essentially fats. These guys are generally known as essential fatty acids because the body cannot make them so they need to be obtained through food. However, looking at all omega-3 and omega-6 fatty acids in this way is a little simplistic, because there are different forms of omega-3 and omega-6. You see, they both come in short and long chains. This is not Biochemistry 101, so I will try to keep this as simple as possible, but I just want you to know that they are not all the same—as is the story with saturated fats, they too are not all the same.

Both omega-3 and omega-6 fatty acid chains come in different lengths. They are found in plants and animals (mostly meats and oils) and we need them for normal body metabolism and good health. Below is a table outlining the various forms of omega-3 and omega-6 fatty acids and the foods that contain them.

TYPE OF FATTY ACID	PRIMARY FOOD SOURCE
Omega-6 short chain (linoleic acid)	seeds, nuts, grains, legumes and vegetable and seed oils, such as soybean oil and corn oil.
Omega-6 long chain (arachidonic acid)	Meat, some fish and eggs.
Omega-3 short chain (alpha-linolenic acid)	Flax seeds, chia seeds, certain vegetable oils and some leafy greens.

TYPE OF FATTY ACID	PRIMARY FOOD SOURCE
Omega-3 long chain (EPA and DHA)	Oily, cold-water fish such as tuna, sardines, anchovies, salmon and in algae.

Both omega-3 and omega-6 fatty acids are needed for good health, but we need them in the correct balance as both fats compete for space in our bodies and it is this balance that has changed drastically over the years. Generally speaking, omega-3 fatty acids are considered anti-inflammatory (the good guys) and omega-6 fatty acids are considered pro-inflammatory (sometimes the bad guys).

To maintain good health, the correct ratio when eating these fatty acids should be about 1 to 2 omega-6s for every 1 omega-3. It is estimated that in today's society we have ratios of around 15 to 17 omega-6s to every 1 omega-3, and that's being conservative. I am sure there are higher omega-6 levels being consumed out there! From a dietary perspective, this imbalance is caused by the over consumption of grains, seed and vegetable oils, processed foods, baked goods and snacks—all of which are high in short-chain omega-6 fatty acids.

Let's use soybean oil as an example. I have chosen the soybean because it is one of the most highly processed and widely used crops to provide oil and proteins. In 2004, world soybean production reached 217 million metric tonnes! Soybeans are used (as an emulsification agent or binder) to make everything from baked goods, flours and meat products to cosmetics and pharmaceuticals. It even has industrial applications and is used in roof coatings and car-engine protectants. You just can't get away from the stuff! And the thing is, it has a horrible omega-6 to omega-3 ratio (soybean oil has about 51 per cent omega-6 to 7 per cent omega-3) and contains some of the most highly allergenic proteins.

Below is a table listing some of the processed products made from soybean oil (and processed oils are far more widespread in your diet through processed food than you may think).

SOYBEAN OIL

Cooking oils

Coffee whiteners (creamers)

Margarine

Salad oils

Whipped toppings

Shortenings

Butter substitutes

Chocolate

Lolly coatings (candy)

Salad dressings

Lollies (candy)

Chocolate

Mayonnaise

Frozen desserts

Emulsifying agents

Spreads

Pastry filling

Dietary supplements

Cheese dips

Gravy mixes

Excess omega-6 causes more prolonged inflammation, constricts the airways and blood vessels, increases blood clotting, reduces circulation and increases pain sensitivity. Excess omega-6 consumption is associated with many lifestyle conditions such as increased cardiovascular disease, diabetes, obesity, arthritis, joint pain, asthma, allergies, metabolic syndrome (also known as syndrome X) and other metabolic conditions—the list goes on!

I will cover more about omega-6 and its implications with the inflammatory pathways in the body in Chapter 7, but I want you to start being aware of the amounts of omega-6 in your diet and where it is coming from.

Allergies

The World Health Organization ranks allergies (generally food allergies, eczema, asthma and allergic rhinitis) as the fourth most common global chronic disease, with the highest rates in developed countries (including the big four: Australia, New Zealand, the United Kingdom and the United States). The interesting thing is, as developing countries adopt a more 'Westernised lifestyle' including more processed 'Western foods', so too are their rates escalating. Data from Australia (a country with one of the highest rates of food allergies in the world) is showing a ten-fold increase in referrals to specialists—not the sort of statistics to be proud of.

Young children are the people most commonly affected by food allergies, and many allergies that were once seen as 'childhood allergies' that the child would eventually grow out of are now persisting through to adulthood. Also, a natural progression from food-related allergies to respiratory allergies (such as asthma), known as the 'allergic march', is becoming more prominent. Although children suffer the highest rates of allergies, it has also been shown that allergies can run in the family. New research is showing that, over several generations, changes in gene expression is occurring due to environmental pressures, which may amplify heritable disease risk. That is, children may be becoming more susceptible to allergies because their genes have been weakened by the toxins that have been passed down from previous generations.

The big-ticket food triggers still seem to be wheat, cow's milk, soy, peanuts, corn and eggs. The issue with these foods is that due to our industrialised food processing, they are in everything! Even if they are not actually listed in the product itself, how often do you see 'may contain traces of nuts' on its packaging? It's because whatever you were eating was manufactured in the same place that millions of other products are made.

The other issue is with food development itself and, again, I will use the soybean as an example, but similarities can be seen in wheat, corn and dairy processing. Since the 1960s, soy has been used to create a variety of 'food-like substances', but it is also one of the most allergenic substances out there. You can get soy flour, soy flakes, soy grits, soy protein concentrate and isolate (a highly concentrated refined protein made from soy). It is also used in the emulsification, foaming and binding of food products and is added to everything from baby formula, cookies, pizza and meat products to ice cream, soups, sauces, noodles, breakfast cereals—the list goes on. It is also added to animal feed.

So the challenging thing is, if you are eating all these sorts of foods and you have allergies, how would you even know where to start to try to establish exactly *what* you are allergic to? Keep in mind that we have not even touched on the environmental ways you can come in contact with soy. It is used in hair and skin products and even auto-care and building materials. You just can't get away from this stuff!

What about adults who develop a food allergy, or adults and children with food intolerance?

True food allergies and food intolerances are very different; it's a complex subject. A true food allergy is an immune response and can have very sudden and severe symptoms, such as anaphylaxis. A food intolerance can be delayed and very subtle, and is caused by reactions to food additives or natural chemicals in foods. Reactions can manifest as skin disorders, headaches, sleep disturbances, behavioural problems and intestinal upset (such as bloating, flatulence and cramps).

Food intolerances and allergies are also on the increase due to a decline in microbial exposure and an increased pro-inflammatory diet. A perfect example of how to develop increased intestinal permeability! (See Chapter 6 to find out all about that.)

Excess salt in the diet

I always like to say to people that it is not the salt that you put on your food you should be worried about. That is not the issue when we are talking about excess salt in the diet. It is the hidden salt in processed food products that does the harm. Salt (sodium chloride) is one of the most widely used additives in food manufacturing and processing because of its low cost and myriad uses. It is used as a preservative, to 'hold' water in meat products, as an antimicrobial agent, and as a flavour enhancer.

The average intake of salt by adults in developed countries is around 7g per day, which, for example, is nearly double the maximum recommended dietary allowance (RDA) in Australia. Your body does need salt—it needs a delicate balance of sodium (salt) and potassium to regulate blood pressure via the kidneys, but an excess of salt throws out this balance. Excess salt causes the kidneys to retain more water which, in turn, increases total blood volume causing your blood pressure to go up (hypertension). Hypertension is linked to an increased risk of cardiovascular disease. On top of this, some people react to sodium with symptoms such as headaches, asthma and skin irritations.

Additives and preservatives

This one is another Pandora's box of potential issues. Food additives and preservatives have come under a lot of scrutiny over the years and I wish they would come under fire more often.

Additives are added to food to enhance flavour or colour (mainly for aesthetic appeal), as these 'food-like substances' would otherwise be undesirable to eat according to a study by Berzas et al. Nice! Does that sound like something that would be good for you? I think not. Franken-food, anyone?

Food additives are mainly used to provide a 'technological function'—to improve the colour, taste, texture or appearance of food, as well as to preserve and to prevent rancidity. So, in essence, they are there to make the product last longer on the supermarket shelf and to appear more attractive to the buyer.

Where it all gets a bit murky is in the wording of ingredients on packaged foods. For example, you will often see the words 'free from artificial flavours and preservatives'. Well, arsenic is natural and so is petroleum, but does that mean you want to consume them? There are many 'natural' substances in the world that are not so good for our health. Some food additives fall into this category, especially for people with a sensitivity to them. A package might have on the ingredients list 'natural colour—caramel (150)'. This is actually produced synthetically by treating carbohydrates in the presence of other substances, such as ammonia or sulphur dioxide—a very crude use of the word 'natural', if you ask me.

Products that commonly include food additives are tinned foods, packaged foods, margarines, processed meats, cheeses, breads, lollies and sweets, bottled drinks, dried fruits—pretty much anything that comes in a packet or can at the supermarket. Even fresh food does not escape—fresh fruit is often coated with propylene glycol to help retain moisture and increase shelf life. Some nasty preservatives and additives to look out for include the following.

Monosodium Glutamate (MSG)

MSG has no taste of its own and no nutritional value; it is purely there to enhance or modify the flavour of foods. It has been linked to a wide range of adverse health effects including heart palpitations, asthma, rashes and migraines. MSG is sometimes listed on food packaging as 621 or other closely related flavour enhances such as 620, 622, 623, 624 and 635. Hydrolysed vegetable protein is also used as an alternative to MSG, and can have the same adverse effects as MSG.

Aspartame

Aspartame (listed on packaging as 951) was first approved for use in Australia in 1981, as a way of sweetening products without the additional calories you would get from sugar, which is why it is often found in 'diet' foods and drinks. Surprisingly, it is found in many other foods such as rice crackers and sausages and instant coffee. It has been linked to headaches, migraines, fatigue, rashes, depression and many other adverse health effects.

Sulphites

Sulphites can also be found listed under the numbers 220–228. They are generally used to keep foods looking fresh and colourful. They have been shown to trigger asthma attacks and are linked to gastric irritation, rashes and diarrhoea. I buy dried fruit that is sulphite free; it is much browner and not so pretty looking, but at least I know it won't hurt me!

Artificial colours

Most of us are aware of the link between artificial colours and hyperactivity, but did you know that many are also suspected carcinogens (cancer-causing substances)? What is also scary is that according to Julie Eady, author of *Additive Alert: Your guide to safer shopping* (2006), there are colours that are banned in other countries that are still allowed in Australia. These include: amaranth (123), Food Green (142), Brilliant Black (151), Carbon Black (153) and Brown HT (155). Artificial colours don't just hide in lollies and treat foods—tartrazine (a yellow food colour) is found in some fruit juices.

***

Additives have been linked to a host of health conditions but most notably childhood behavioural disorders such as attention deficit hyperactivity disorder (ADHD) and attention deficit disorder (ADD). A study by Bateman et al. at the University of Southampton showed that tartrazine was linked to hyperactivity in children as well as restlessness, sleep disturbances and other behavioural changes—even with levels lower than concentrations used in foods. In a study by Kashanian and Zeidali, which looked at the prolonged used of this colour dye in rats, a significant increase to DNA damage in colon cells, hepatic and renal changes and an increased number of gastric mucosa lymphocytes was reported. This indicates that there was possibly damage to the gut wall, promoting inflammation and the activation of the immune system (hello gut damage and increased intestinal permeability again!).

The issue with additives and preservatives is the cumulative effect—the adding up of many, many, many small amounts. Then there is the 5 per cent loophole in the Food Standards Code for Australia and New Zealand. If the amount of the additive or preservative is less than 5 per cent for that 'food', it does not have to be listed on the label. Another way you can keep getting your many, many small amounts!

Can you see a bit of a pattern here? So, what is the easiest way to avoid all these issues about safe and unsafe processed food? Don't eat it. If you can't pronounce something on the label unless you went to chemistry class—don't eat it. If the food has too many numbers on the label—don't eat it. If it doesn't go mouldy and is not biodegradable—don't eat it. If it is a highly allergenic, anti-nutrient food—don't eat it (I will explain what the anti-nutrients are in grains and legumes in Chapter 3).

Eating real, whole food is one of the easiest, most cost-effective ways you can practise preventative health for you and your family.

How is it that our bodies don't identify inappropriate foods as foreign?

Well, the truth is that all food is technically foreign to the body (until we digest it efficiently into its components and reintegrate them into our own bodies). However, when it comes to signs of unsuitability, it often does give us signs, yet we often don't notice them (until we know what to look for, that is).

One of the primary signs of your body being at odds with the food you eat is the disturbance we see to the metabolism (especially those from refined foods), such as fluctuations to body weight and blood sugar/energy levels.

Secondary mechanisms by which our diet shows signs of unsuitability to our body relate to the nutritional deficiencies we see hinder so many of our basic body processes. As a result of food depleted of essential nutrients being presented to the body to simply tick all the 'caloric boxes' (and therefore tweak all our instincts of salivating palatability), without actually delivering the real nutrient payload, our evolutionary instincts have developed to associate with these cues. So we see our body's needs for essential nourishment go unmet and are therefore left unable to stave off many of the increasingly prevalent modern chronic diseases (that have nutrient deficiencies at their heart).

Beyond these metabolic aspects, however, is the very significant consideration of food allergies and the immune system's ability to identify specific food components as foreign enough to mount an attack/defence to them (when it comes to the immune system, attack certainly is considered the best form of defence).

It is sometimes hard to say whether this response is appropriate or not, given the fact that all food components are originally foreign to the body, and thus even 'whole' foods, just as much as 'processed' foods can be the targets of attack. Optimum digestion (sufficient stomach acid, bile production and digestive enzymes) therefore remains our primary defence against intact food components (mostly protein fragments) being able to make their way into the bloodstream to be attacked by the immune system. The abovementioned nutritional deficiencies and disturbances to normal metabolism can each play a role in impairing efficient digestion and so a vicious circle of each contributing to the other can emerge. All the more reason to optimise our digestion and eat real food.

When we have insufficient digestive ability to process certain food components, the classic symptoms of inflammation and rejection, such as abdominal pain and diarrhoea, often follow. However, the symptoms of all types of food sensitivity can be very tricky to pin down. Partly due to the many varied mechanisms with which we can react to foods (some can appear as joint pains, some as skin rashes and others even as behavioural changes etc.), we usually need some assistance to pin these down.

Clinically, beyond a good diet history and food rotation plan, we often need food antibody assessments to help us identify the foods our immune system is most reactive to. Namely two antibodies—IgA and IgG—need to be assessed for a more comprehensive assessment of delayed food sensitivities (simply via a quick blood spot sample that can be taken in a clinic by a trained nutritionist or naturopath). This is because most food sensitivity reactions are delayed (up to three to four days after consuming the offending food!) and some (IgA) give little to no symptomatic feedback at all, despite playing a key role in the formation of further subsequent inflammation by leaving the digestive tract increasingly vulnerable to degeneration, infection and further allergen sensitisation.

Assessing IgA/IgG food antibodies can therefore also provide a great indication of how much digestive inflammation/permeability is present within the gut (otherwise referred to as 'leaky gut'), when many elevations are revealed by testing.

So, the key issue here is inflammation, and beyond its triggers, the body's biggest determinant as to the likelihood and strength of an inflammatory response comes down to the balance of omega-6 and omega-3 within our body tissues, which is yet another diet-determined factor. A highly processed modern (omega-6 excessive) diet tends to skew towards the highly inflammatory side, even when free from any major food sensitivities, but especially if we have any of the ever-increasingly common food sensitivities discussed here.

So, clinically I would recommend testing both IgA and IgG food specific antibodies (to about 100 foods each) as well as the balance of omega-6 and omega-3 fats in your body via a Red Blood Cell Lipid Profile test, both of which can be sampled via a simple blood spot test, by a functionally trained doctor, nutritionist or naturopath.

—Warren Maginn, functional clinical nutritionist

CHAPTER 3

What is all the fuss about grains, legumes and dairy?

So, we learnt in Chapter 2 that according to the World Health Organization, our rates of food allergies are skyrocketing and the most common culprits include dairy, wheat and soy. Is that surprising to me? No, not really. It has been recognised in naturopathic medicine for a long time that compounds in these foods can cause health issues.

Now, depending on how much you like to geek out, you might want to further investigate these anti-nutrient compounds. I am just going to give you a brief explanation behind some of the mechanisms causing food allergies and inflammation, so you can understand why these foods can negatively impact our health.

Grains and legumes

So, what is all the fuss about? Well, these guys have some compounds in them—natural toxins and gut-irritating proteins—that may not be so good for our health. These compounds can interfere with the absorption of nutrients and cause disruption to your digestion leading to inflammation, nutritional deficiencies and possibly more severe chronic inflammatory conditions such as leaky-gut syndrome.

Plants naturally want to continue their life cycle—to be able to grow and reproduce so as to ensure the survival of their species. In order to be able to do this, they have some defence mechanisms in place to ward off the predators that eat them (yes, that includes us). Essentially, these mechanisms are geared towards either the survival of the reproductive part of the plant passing through the digestive tract intact (of the animal that eats it) so that it can germinate and grow again, or causing so much intestinal distress from eating the plant that the animal won't want to eat that plant or seed again. Fun times!

Signs and symptoms of intestinal distress can include bloating, gas and general gastrointestinal upset, but many symptoms such as inflammation and vitamin or mineral deficiencies may go unrecognised for a period of time. And some of the more serious conditions that these guys are implicated with include infertility, osteoporosis, autoimmune diseases and mental conditions. So, what are some of these compounds?

Lectins

- Lectins are found in nearly all plants but are most notably in grains, legumes, nuts, dairy and nightshade plants (eggplant, tomatoes, potatoes).

- Lectins bind to surface proteins in the digestive tract. This can impair the function of the gut wall leading to increased gastrointestinal permeability (leaky gut), reduced enzyme activity, reduced nutrient digestion and absorption, gut bacteria imbalances and impaired immune functioning.

Phytates/Phytic acid

- Phytates are found in grains, legumes, nuts and seeds and bind with the minerals in these foods, forming indigestible compounds. This means the calcium, iron, zinc and magnesium found in these foods cannot be absorbed efficiently by your body.

- Zinc and magnesium deficiency are two of the most common mineral deficiencies that many practitioners see. Depletion of our soil and the high consumption of grains could potentially be driving these deficiencies.

Saponins

- Saponins have foamy, soap-like characteristics and are bitter. They actually have the ability to punch holes in the membranes of the cells that make up the brush border (villi) in your small intestine.

- Saponins can be very irritating on the gut and promote an immune response.

- Saponins are found in pseudo-grains such as quinoa, but are sometimes partially removed before the commercial sale of food.

Gluten

- Gluten is the main protein structure (a combination of gliadins and glutenins) found in wheat, rye, barley and oats.

- Wheat is one of the most commonly consumed cereals worldwide, yet many people (estimated above 80 per cent) have a subclinical sensitivity to gluten and the protein is poorly digested.

- Gluten causes damage to your gastrointestinal tract and other parts of your body through the promotion of systemic inflammation and increased intestinal permeability, and it activates an immune response. Chronic inflammation has been linked to autoimmune diseases, heart disease, neuropathy, depression and schizophrenia.

- In the past 50 years, there has been a massive surge in new gluten-related disorders coming to light.

The effects of many of these compounds are dose dependant, meaning that if you only eat a very small amount, infrequently, you may not suffer any adverse consequences. But this is assuming you have perfect gut integrity, which none of us does.

It is also worth noting that proper preparation of these foods can inactivate some of the toxins. Traditional preparation processes such as soaking, sprouting, cooking or fermenting seeds or legumes can inactivate some of these toxins. So, should you eat grains and legumes?

Gluten-containing grains

- I believe that the cons far outweigh the pros. There is nothing in gluten-containing grains that you can't get in a more bio-available form from vegetables, fruit and meats.

- Gluten-containing grains, such as wheat, contain opioid peptides, which actually makes eating foods containing gluten addictive.

Gluten-free grains and pseudo-grains

- Caution should be considered here as gluten-free grains and pseudo-grains have many of the same concerns as gluten-containing grains, and they are foods that people regularly consume in excess. Making sure that you have good gut health (no leaky gut) is essential before considering the introduction of these foods. It is also worth noting that these foods can potentially be eaten in excess and accompany emotional eating. You should understand your food triggers before deciding if these foods are right for you.

Legumes

- The anti-nutrients in most legumes can be inactivated through soaking and cooking, although some of the lectins may remain.

- Only consider possibly reintroducing legumes into your diet after you have done an elimination protocol and spent some time healing the gut (outlined in Chapter 13).

- I would still strongly suggest avoiding soy and peanuts. They are two of the most allergenic foods available. You are hard pressed to get your hands on nongenetically modified soy these days and it is a known endocrine disrupter. There is nothing good about these two!

What about potatoes?

Potatoes contain glycoalkaloids, which is concentrated mostly in the skin. A majority of the glycoalkaloids are removed through peeling the skin, but some remains. These compounds can be problematic to people with a leaky gut, so again, proceed with caution.

What about rice?

In their book *Perfect Health Diet,* Paul and Shou-Ching Jaminet state that white rice contains minimal toxins after cooking. A couple of toxins found in rice include phytin (a phytate) and trypsin inhibitors (trypsin is an enzyme that breaks down protein), but most of these are denatured during the cooking process. As is the case with all grains, most of the vitamins and minerals are contained in the bran (the outer covering). While you may think eating bran is a good thing, this is also where most of the problem proteins and anti-nutrients exist. This is why eating white rice is less problematic than eating brown rice because the protein found in the bran of rice has been found to provoke an immune-system response.

What about nuts and seeds?

These guys also contain phytic acid, but 'activating' your nuts and seeds will reduce the amounts found in these foods. Soaking them in water overnight begins the sprouting process, which reduces the phytic acid and makes the nutrients more bio-available. However, nuts and seeds are still foods that should be eaten in very small amounts.

Dairy

Dairy is one of the top five foods linked to allergies—a lot of people have issues tolerating dairy. The news with dairy is all pretty much the same as with wheat.

- Dairy contains the proteins casein and whey, and the milk sugar lactose.

- Many people are not only sensitive to the lactose, but they also have issues digesting the milk proteins. This can result in an unhealthy balance of gut bacteria, leaky-gut syndrome, increased inflammation, diarrhoea, bloating, etc.

- Dairy also contains casomorphins—opioid peptides found in the casein. Dairy with a high proportion of casein (e.g. cheese) can be addictive.

- Pasteurisation damages milk proteins and may reduce their nutritional quality and affect their functional properties. Thermal damage to milk may also affect calcium availability.

- It is illegal in most countries to sell raw dairy because of the potential for bacterial contamination. Raw dairy contains lactase (the enzyme that breaks down lactose) and it is this enzyme that many adults lack. This makes raw milk sometimes more tolerable to people sensitive to dairy.

- What about A2 milk? In the past few years there has been a lot of talk about the differences between A1 and A2 cow's milk. Each type of milk contains its own beta-casein protein: A1 beta-casein protein and A2 beta-protein. It is the genetic variation at the 67th position of a single amino acid on these two protein chains that is different. The theory is that the active peptide BCM7 is released during the digestion of A1 milk, but not with A2. The BCM7 peptide has been linked to type 1 diabetes and even heart disease, but reviews of this research by Truswell state that there is no convincing or even probable evidence of A1 milk having any adverse effect on humans. It is worth considering though that people with impaired digestion or leaky gut (which can be a lot of people) could possibly have issues breaking down the BCM7 peptide and perhaps that is why, anecdotally, many people respond favourably when swapping from A1 to A2 milk.

In the world of dairy, what does seem less problematic to people is dairy fats in the form of heavy cream and butter. The higher the fat content, the lower the levels of the problematic proteins and sugars. You also get the added bonus of good fats such as omega-3 and conjugated linoleic acid (any issues you might have with saturated fats are covered in Chapter 10).

What about calcium?

You might be surprised to know that the calcium you find in dairy is not actually the most bio-available form out there. Greens such as kale and broccoli actually trump dairy for containing calcium in a form your body loves to absorb. Almonds, sunflower seeds and sesame seeds are also good choices for non-dairy calcium. Another is bone broth—a Paleo staple! You do not have to consume dairy in order to get your recommended daily intake of calcium.

What is the benefit of eating dairy if it does nothing but drive pro-inflammatory conditions in your body? It will impede your absorption of not only the calcium you are trying to get from it, but also your digestion and absorption of EVERYTHING you eat. Not very beneficial!

If you do find that you are able to tolerate some dairy in your diet, make sure that it is from grass-fed cows, how nature intended. A happy, healthy cow will pass on those healthy nutrients to you! But how do you know if the beef you're buying is grass-fed? I recommend buying from a butcher rather than a supermarket, so that you can ask all the relevant questions. Most butchers are happy to have a chat with you, and grass-fed beef is becoming a more popular request. If your butcher does not carry it, they are usually happy to source some for you. When you actually look at grass-fed beef compared to grain-fed, the fat will be a lovely, almost orangey colour. This is from the beta-carotene (vitamin A) the meat contains from the cow eating its natural grass diet.

What about fermented dairy?

Yoghurt and fermented milk drinks, such as kefir, have some benefits due to the fermentation process because some of the lactose and milk proteins have been broken down. Some people who have issues with other forms of dairy can tolerate fermented dairy, but some can't. It is something that you need to try out for yourself and see if you can tolerate it without any adverse reactions. It is also worth noting that the yoghurt should be full fat and pot set, but I cover more about that in Chapter 13.

The main points to remember about eating grains, legumes and dairy are:

- Some, but not all, of these foods can be problematic to many people. It is about seeing what works for your body and what doesn't.

- There are other food choices that you can make that are more nutrient dense and do not have the associated problematic compounds—so why wouldn't you choose to consume something that is potentially less harmful?

- Some of these foods contain opioid-like compounds, which can make these foods addictive and hard to give up.

- These foods are predominately carbohydrates and are potentially over consumed in large amounts. This is not optimal for our health or our hormonal responses (covered in Chapter 4).

As I mentioned at the beginning of the chapter, this is just a very brief summary of why these foods may not be the best choice for your health. There are many good sources out there where you can find greater in-depth information. Just remember that it is not all about the food. What you eat is just one piece of the puzzle. Your lifestyle also plays a big role in your health, as does whether you suffer from chronic stress or an illness. And although a small amount of one of these foods might not be that bad, it is a cumulative effect of all of these assaults on your defences that causes the bigger health concerns. These foods are not ALL bad. Let's take dairy as an example. Dairy contains good levels of vitamin A, magnesium, zinc, potassium and essential amino acids such as tryptophan. If you can tolerate dairy, include it in your diet, but remember, it does not need to be an all-or-nothing approach. Find out which types of dairy suit you best—whether it be full fat or fermented—and only consume those. It is about being aware that some foods just might be more beneficial for you and that there are other nutrient-dense, less problematic choices.

CHAPTER 4

Out-of-control hormones

Hormones are a big deal. I am not expecting you all to be budding endocrinologists, but I just want you to have an idea about some of the main participants in the 'food' camp when it comes to hormones. It will give you an idea of the sorts of things hormones regulate and what happens when they start to get out of whack. Your hormones work like one big connected network and it is not as easy as A affects B. It's more like A affects B and C disrupts D and causes more E to be released which stops F being produced! It is a very complicated process, so bear with me. Having some understanding about these hormones will further empower you to know how you got to your current state of health and *how* hormones can affect your health for the better or worse.

Hormones are chemical messengers that are released in one part of the body (usually via blood) but regulate the activity in another part of the body (usually by binding to receptors). Most people are familiar with our sex hormones (the likes of testosterone and oestrogen) but there are many more hormones that all have different jobs regulating various things within our body.

> Your hormones work like one big connected network and it is not as easy as A affects B. It's more like A affects B and C disrupts D and causes more E to be released which stops F being produced!

Hormones have a variety of roles, but one of their primary functions is to maintain homeostasis—to keep things in balance and within levels that will keep you out of harm's way (so to speak). When you do things like eat, or not eat, for a period of time, or when you are stressed or are exposed to toxins, hormones are released to deal with that imbalance. For example, the act of eating (even good food) will cause different hormones to be released into the bloodstream and because you have changed the balance of the environment inside your body by the addition of various nutrients and energy, your body needs to figure out what it wants to do with them and how it wants to store them. Let's take a peek at some of the participants in the food camp of hormones!

Leptin

Leptin is a hormone that is primarily produced by adipocytes (fat cells), but also by the skeletal muscle, ovaries, stomach, bone marrow, pituitary gland and liver. Leptin regulates food intake, energy expenditure and glucose and fat metabolism by signalling to the brain information about nutrient status—it is the hormone that signals to the brain that we are 'full' after eating a meal. It also regulates how much energy (fat) we have in storage and when we need to take in more energy.

Higher leptin levels are seen in people with a higher fat content in their body and therefore you would think they have higher satiety levels (not be so hungry), but often in overweight and obese people the reverse is seen. Something called leptin resistance can develop, where the signal given by the leptin to the brain that you are full is lost, so you constantly feel hungry, despite having more than enough stored fat to use as energy.

Leptin levels are generally highest in the evening, which is why you can fall asleep and not be woken up with the midnight munchies. It is quite low in the morning when you wake up, which is when leptin's counter hormone ghrelin is secreted and makes you feel hungry.

The mechanism through which leptin resistance can develop is still the subject of research, but some of the possible reasons for why it happens include: an over consumption of sugary junk foods leading to consistently high blood glucose and triglyceride levels, high C-reactive protein levels (high C-reactive is a protein seen in the bloodstream in response to inflammation) and increased oxidative stress caused by free radicals.

Free radicals are molecules with an unpaired electron, looking to take another electron from another molecule so it can pair up. This 'stealing' of electrons can result in damage to your cells. Free radicals are a product of our body's natural processes, but also come from external factors such as environmental toxins, cigarette smoke and herbicides.

It is also worth noting that bacterial infections such as *Helicobacter pylori* (a bug that can set up camp in your stomach lining and cause ulcers) can impact the expression of both leptin and ghrelin.

Ghrelin

Ghrelin is the only known orexigenic hormone, meaning that it acts as an appetite stimulant. It also decreases energy usage and promotes weight gain. Interestingly, it has been found that ghrelin enhances the intake of palatable food (in particular sugary foods) and is involved in the reward pathway in your brain—increasing the release of the neurotransmitters dopamine and acetylcholine, both of which make you feel reward, arousal, gratification and pleasure. Often people want to keep this pleasurable feeling going, so they seek out more of the palatable food to keep feeding this feeling. It is the same pathway involved with particular drug addictions.

Repeat after me: sleep is the most important thing to me; sleep is the most important thing to me!

When ghrelin is at normal levels and functioning correctly, it does a great job—like all hormones in our body. But what upsets the normal balance of ghrelin levels in your body? Lack of sleep!

Studies have shown that even a single night of sleep deprivation increases ghrelin levels. Not only does lack of sleep increase ghrelin levels, but it decreases leptin levels—a double whammy! You feel like you can't control your eating, you crave sugary foods and you put on weight. You blame yourself and think you have no self-control, but it is not always the case—your body's chemistry could be coming into play!

Chronic sleep deprivation or lack of a good night's sleep is a huge health concern in our society today. Above everything (yep, even food), one of the best things you can do for your health is to make getting a good night's sleep, EVERY NIGHT, a priority.

Repeat after me: *Sleep is the most important thing to me; sleep is the most important thing to me!*

Insulin

Insulin's main jobs are regulating blood sugar levels by facilitating the storage of fats, carbohydrates and proteins into the cells, and speeding up the conversion of glucose to glycogen (known as glycogenesis). Insulin is a building hormone mainly linked to carbohydrate consumption; think of it as a 'stockpiler' of goodies. It is released by the beta cells in the pancreas in response to a rise in blood sugar levels, such as when you have just eaten something, the nutrients have been broken down, and have now entered the bloodstream.

> Our blood sugar levels like to remain pretty constant ... Chronically high blood sugar levels are dangerous, as are low blood sugar levels—our body likes balance.

Our blood sugar levels like to remain pretty constant and when a rise is noticed, the pancreas releases insulin to help restore the balance. Chronically high blood sugar levels are dangerous, as are low blood sugar levels—our body likes balance. Chronically raised blood sugar levels can cause damage to various organs in the body—the pancreas, liver and brain to name a few!

When you have raised blood sugar levels, your body tries to deal with it by storing as much glucose as it can in your muscles and liver, and then the rest is converted to fat and triglycerides anything it can do to bring those blood sugars back down to normal levels.

Stress and cortisol play a part in this as well. Cortisol inhibits insulin production, because it wants glucose to stay in the blood to be used as immediate energy. It thinks you need that energy right away because you are going to have to run from a bear ('fight or flight' and bears are covered in Chapter 5). Therefore, cortisol leads to higher blood sugar levels, which lead to higher insulin, which leads to higher cortisol and the cycle continues. Chronically high cortisol is implicated in insulin resistance, along with continually flooding the body with insulin due to nutrient-poor/high-carbohydrate food consumption, so that the body does not 'hear' the signal anymore. Tumour necrosis factor alpha (TNF-a) and Interleukin-6 (IL-6) are two inflammatory cytokines (inflammatory markers) that are also implicated in insulin resistance, showing again that systemic inflammation affects all areas of your health.

Glucagon

Glucagon is your counter buddy to insulin; it is released from pancreatic alpha cells in response to lowered blood sugar levels. It likes to take the 'stockpile' that insulin has been storing and distribute it for energy use. It raises blood sugar levels through forming glucose from other nutrients in the liver (a process called gluconeogenesis) and converting glycogen to glucose (glycogenolysis—remember those words for your next game of Scrabble). It is also responsible for the release of fat to be used as energy. This is when your body starts to tap into its fat resources to keep you going, which is a good thing.

Cortisol also stimulates glucagon into action, because in 'fight or flight' you're going to need energy, right? So, cortisol bumps glucagon into action to make some fuel available for use.

Good glucagon release is only available when insulin is not around. If you are permanently using carbohydrates as your primary fuel source and insulin is always working away in the background, glucagon will never be able to get to do its thing.

So, is eating carbohydrates a bad thing? No, of course not! We need them in our diet. However, eating too many carbs and the wrong type of carbs does not let this ebb and flow happen between insulin and glucagon and you are always 'stockpiling' (putting on excess weight) and never using this energy. Having a proper balance between the two also allows for nice smooth blood sugar levels and no blood sugar spikes, followed by the notorious crash afterwards.

What are two of the best ways to allow glucagon to do its thing? Glucagon is stimulated by exercise or through a rise in blood amino acids (protein) when blood sugars are kept low (e.g. eating a meal that mainly contains protein).

Cortisol

Cortisol is covered in more detail in Chapter 5, but as a hormone, it is part of your normal sleep-and-wake cycle and is one of the key players in the body's stress response. Stressors of any kind can cause cortisol to be released. Chronically high levels of cortisol cause high blood pressure, high blood sugar levels, impaired immune function, digestive issues and inflammation, which is why it is important to reduce any sources of stress in your life. Junk food, sugary foods and drinks such as coffee and energy drinks also cause cortisol to be released.

How does cortisol affect all our other hormones?

As is about to be discussed in Chapter 5, cortisol is a crucial stress hormone with numerous impacts. These cannot be summarised in one chapter because they are so far-reaching to the body. Every system in the human body requires cortisol for harmonious function and any imbalances in its production will have profound and widespread effects.

In particular, one of the primary impacts of excessive cortisol production to the rest of our steroid (cholesterol-based) hormones is that they will each inevitably get less of a share of the basic cholesterol starting material they require and will subsequently suffer reduced production. This is especially true for women, and reduced progesterone production (when the body finds cortisol production more of a priority) unfortunately results in an imbalance of progesterone with oestrogen otherwise known as 'oestrogen dominance'. Oestrogen dominance has a whole raft of metabolic effects associated with it and is, in fact, one of the primary drivers behind some of the most common diseases relating to female reproductive tissues (the breasts, ovaries, uterus, etc.) and can be responsible for period irregularities. Men are similarly affected by reductions in their testosterone levels as a result of high cortisol production.

So, we find that unless we address stress, not only will our adrenal and thyroid glands suffer, but so will our steroid 'gender' hormones. Keeping in mind that these gender hormones are responsible for much of our optimum and defining function as both men and women (i.e. oestrogen, testosterone, progesterone, etc.) we can start to see how hard it might be to maintain our own personal 'optimum' state of being when subjected to prolonged stress.

The most comprehensive method for assessing all cholesterol-based hormones and their intermediate metabolites (to offer insights into the reasons for any imbalances that are found) would be a 24-hour Urinary Hormone Profile. This will not only show all major (and many minor) male and female hormones, but also adrenal hormones associated with the regulation of blood sugar (gluco-corticoids), mineral balance (mineral-corticoids) and, of course, cortisol (over a full circadian cycle), giving a very comprehensive insight into the current distribution of hormone production from cholesterol.

Much of the action of the adrenal 'stress' hormones (adrenaline and cortisol) relates to the management of energy utilisation (both its release and storage) in the body, since one of the primary roles of these hormones is to mobilise the resources that will enable us to fulfil a demand placed on us. The thyroid gland, however, is the main regulator of the rate of cellular energy usage around the body and so we see a certain amount of 'cross-talk' between the thyroid and adrenal glands in effectively managing this energy economy.

This is because the thyroid, adrenal and reproductive organs are all inextricably linked, both directly and indirectly—especially via their shared orchestration through the hypothalamus and pituitary control glands in the brain. This means that changes to the brain and even perceptions can alter the symphony of signals coordinating each of them and have profound effects on our hormones (yes, how we think and feel can affect our hormones and, in turn, our hormones can affect how we feel). Just another set of interconnected systems within us, to be harmonised at both ends of the spectrum, to bring about happiness and harmony.

—Warren Maginn, functional clinical nutritionist

CHAPTER 5

Stress, stress and more stress!

Stress ... we all know about it and we all talk about 'being stressed' at some stage, perhaps even every day! But what I would like to do in this chapter is make you aware of some of the 'stressors' you may have in your life you may not be aware of and what stress is physiologically doing to your body (what effect it is having on your body). Don't get me wrong, a little bit of stress is a good thing; it is what you need to 'get things done' and it is a good motivator. It is when our stresses take over, are continuous, or are too extreme that we run into problems. The key is to recognise what your individual stressors are and then better manage your response to them.

One thing I always do with my clients is to spend a lot of time talking about their stress. You would be surprised how many people think that on a scale of one to ten (one being low stress and ten being high stress) they are actually lower on the stress scale than they are in reality—until I start to point out all the potential areas of 'not so common' stress.

Generally speaking, I like to group stress into emotional/psychological and physical.

Emotional/psychological stressors can include: relationships, mortgage (financial) payments, work, anxiety, fear, frustration, lack of social interaction, low self-esteem, perfectionism and your perception of it.

Physical stressors can include: lack of sleep (such a big issue in today's society), exercise (yes, because exercise causes a stress response in the body), environmental toxins, chronic infections, eating on the run, allergen exposure, alcohol, caffeine, smoking, nutritional deficiencies, even training a new dog (okay, I may have thrown that one in because I am doing it right now ... but trust me, it is causing me stress!).

How we perceive the stressor also plays a big part. How you look at the world also plays a physiological role in how you react to stress. Do you see the world through eyes of fear and anxiety or through the eyes of gratitude and appreciation? Think about all the potential stressors in your life; are there more than you first thought?

QUICK STRESS QUIZ ANSWER YES OR NO TO THE FOLLOWING QUESTIONS.

Do you find it difficult to fall asleep at night or do you wake frequently?	Yes	No
Do you have cravings, especially for sugary foods?	Yes	No
Do you suffer from niggly health issues (frequent colds, headaches, allergies)?	Yes	No

Do you use devices such as laptops, tablets, smart phones or watch TV right up to bedtime or use these devices in bed?	Yes	No
Do you have a hard time quietening your mind at bedtime?	Yes	No
Do you do high-intensity exercise more than four times per week?	Yes	No
Do you need stimulants (coffee, tea, energy drinks) to get through the day?	Yes	No
Do you generally feel fatigued?	Yes	No
Are your meals generally consumed on the run or in front of the TV?	Yes	No
Do daily stresses really anger or emotionally upset you (bad drivers, supermarket queues)?	Yes	No
Do you have financial worries?	Yes	No
Do you catch up with friends less than once a month?	Yes	No

If you have circled 'Yes' more than four times, you should be doing more to reduce the stress in your life!

Acute and chronic stress

We need to differentiate here between acute and chronic stress. Firstly, our stress response is there for a reason and it works damn well, a little too well. When we are faced with a difficult or stressful situation, our body goes into what's called a 'fight or flight' response, which goes back to our ancestral hunter–gatherer days. You see, whenever there was a perceived threat, let's say coming into contact with a big bear or something—you had to be ready to either put your fists up and 'fight' or get nimble with your feet and be ready to take 'flight' and run. We generally don't have bears chasing us these days, but the response is still the same in our body. Our body has the same 'fight or flight' response to all of the stressors listed above—relationship issues, worries about money or a work deadline.

This kind of stress response is meant be short-lived (acute), but in today's world people are suffering from so much stress that this response is happening for extended periods of time, if not all the time, and people are suffering from chronic stress as a result.

What are some of the consequences of persistent and ongoing stress?

This is where we see what is often called the 'Generalised Adaptation Syndrome' (as it was first described by Hans Seyle, the 'father of stress research' way back in 1936). Seyle observed how the body would respond to any external biological source of stress with a predictable biological pattern, in an attempt to restore the body's own internal balance and equilibrium (to maintain survival in ever-changing conditions).

His theory described 'stress' as a major cause of disease, and explained how chronic stress causes long-term biochemical changes within the body. He noted hormonal changes induced by stressors to the body as being sufficient to alter normal metabolism, and determined that we each have a finite supply of 'adaptive energy' with which to withstand stress, and that this amount invariably declines with continuous exposure/demand. (Which sounds a lot like what we refer to as 'functional reserve' within the practice of Functional Medicine.)

Now, it must be noted here that whatever was true in 1936 can only be considered more so today in the context of our modern lifestyles, and has in fact been the primary mechanism with which we have ensured our survival throughout the millennia, from the cave to the corner shop. It goes to the heart of what it means to be human, and thus it pays for us to understand it to a sufficient degree to observe the impact various stressors have on us and our lives, as well as how to address them and the implications of having them continue unresolved for prolonged periods of time. (Tip: the key word here is 'unresolved'.)

The three stages of the Generalised Adaptation Syndrome that your body consistently undertakes to regain its stability in response to any given stressor/s are as follows.

1. 'Alarm' (involving the short-term activation of the HPA axis, the sympathetic nervous system and the adrenal glands that results in a predominantly adrenaline and then cortisol-driven hormonal response, to mobilise energy resources to

accommodate the demands of that acute demand/threat). It is important to note that this stage involves a certain degree of collateral damage, most notably from the high oxidative burden brought about by the elevated blood sugar reserves mobilised by these hormones, and so if this energy is not actually expended through physical exertion (as was intended within the 'flight or fight' response) then the risk factors for heart disease, diabetes and many common modern conditions escalates.

2. The second phase of the response to stress then progresses to 'Resistance', where the body is expecting any momentary threats to have now been resolved and it can begin restoring homeostasis, regeneration and repair. However, a certain amount of sustained cortisol production might be required to maintain resistance to a demand that is ongoing and not fully resolved. Note that even when a momentary stress IS resolved and stress hormones DO return to baseline levels at this stage, our adaptive energy reserve has not yet recovered and we may have reduced defences at this point. Therefore, problems arise when we enter into (or remain within) the Alarm stage too often or for too long, and therefore begin to bypass this second stage and progress to the third stage—'exhaustion'.

3. The third phase in the response to stress therefore relates to the progression to 'Exhaustion', where your 'adaptive energy supply' has been

depleted. Often referred to as 'overload', 'burnout' or 'adrenal fatigue', and is characterised by persistently elevated stress hormones that ultimately begin to dwindle to low levels that offer little adaptive capacity to change, threat or exertion. This will have far-reaching effects on multiple organ systems of the body, most notably the nervous system and at this point, apart from severe fatigue and limited stamina, thinking and memory are often impaired as well as an increased risk of progression towards generalised anxiety and/or depression. Dysfunctions to the autonomic nervous system can also precipitate impacts on the immune system, and has been implicated within chronic infections and rheumatoid arthritis to name a few.

Fear not (for that would be ironic), because with both awareness and empowerment, we can chose an alternate path. In fact, interestingly, some studies have shown that placing a 'positive context' or better still a positive resolution to any momentary stress actually has beneficial effects, perhaps like a muscle, by encouraging us to store more reserves for future such demands and enable us to get better at 'rising to challenges', whereas unresolved stressors or ones that resulted in a perception of 'failure' show more of the negative impacts described above.

These stressors we've discussed so far have related predominantly to 'psychological' stressors. What about the 'biochemical' stressors that we are exposed to on a daily basis? These include toxins, infections, allergens etc. and can each put the exact same type of demands on our cortisol production as the psychological stressors, and so can deplete our metabolic reserves simply from excessive exposure and so, consequently, they also need to be addressed (noting that we often have little to no direct symptomatic feedback as to their presence, despite still being straws upon the 'camel's back').

So, any adrenal preservation/recovery program should not forget to include accurate assessments of these often underestimated and overlooked 'biochemical' stressors. I would recommend testing for metal toxicity via an accurate Hair or Urine Mineral Analysis, as well as food sensitivities via an IgA/IgG blood spot test, and conducting a Comprehensive Stool Analysis (CSA) to assess the balance of bacteria/parasites in the gut in order to make accurate and appropriate assessments of these highly noteworthy burdens with a functionally trained naturopath, nutritionist or doctor.

Key tips:

• It would be great to get physical exercise and maintain fitness for general health overall, but if this is too much for you and your lifestyle, then AT LEAST when you feel the 'fright' or 'pressure' coursing through your veins, go for a run, get to the gym or exert yourself in some way to 'burn off the steam'.

• Make sure your environment supports low cortisol levels; remember that noise stress is a considerable environmental stress—and the right choice of music or ambient sound has been measured to lower cortisol levels.

• Make sure you frame your pressures in a positive way and see what they bring to your life more than perceive what they 'threaten'.

• And lastly and perhaps most importantly, make sure any notable stressors are resolved within a reasonable time frame. Re-evaluate the consequences and appropriateness of long-standing unrelenting pressure to your wellbeing.

Given our finite capacity for energy production/reserve, it becomes apparent that the likelihood of progressing to the 'exhaustion' phase from prolonged and excessive states of 'alarm' (that can be brought about by any or all of the abovementioned factors) is all too common in the modern world. But it is something that those of us now 'in-the-know' might be surprised to know is within our control to address, if we know what to look for and emphasise, to maintain a vibrant life (annoyingly, however, control is perhaps not one of them).

—Warren Maginn, functional clinical nutritionist

'Fight or Flight' and stress hormones

So, what happens when you experience this 'fight or flight' response? Hormones are released in your body in preparation to help you 'fight' or run away from that big damn bear, of course! The main stress hormones involved are cortisol, adrenaline (epinephrine) and noradrenaline (norepinephrine).

Cortisol

Cortisol is released by the adrenal glands in response to stress, but also as a part of your natural circadian rhythm (your sleep-and-wake cycle). This means that it should be highest in the morning (around 6 to 8a.m.) to help you wake up, and then slowly subsides over the course of the day. It then has another peak at around 3 to 4p.m., and then should slowly drop off to negligible levels at night, when another hormone called melatonin kicks in to help you sleep.

Stress causes cortisol to be released (in addition to the above circadian rhythm) to assist your body to deal with the upcoming danger (although in our world that danger might be our mortgage stress, not a bear). Increased levels of cortisol can affect glucose metabolism, blood pressure, insulin release, immune function, digestion and inflammation—not to mention high levels can stop you sleeping at night! Have you ever been anxious, over-thinking something or had caffeine too late in the afternoon and you have been unable to sleep? That is high cortisol levels.

What is the most accurate way to determine your overall stress status, as well as your capacity to withstand it?

Well, this is where you couldn't go past a Diurnal x4 Saliva Cortisol Test. This test simply involves taking a small vial of saliva at four intervals in the day (morning, noon, afternoon and evening) to have the levels of cortisol produced at each of these intervals plotted for you on a graph. The significance of this is in the pattern you produce throughout your day (hence the word 'diurnal' referring to the day portion of your circadian rhythm) and is a great way to assess whether the general balance of your lifestyle is in line with a normal pattern of rise and fall in this time window.

Some people may show general overproduction of cortisol throughout the day. Others may show overproduction in the morning allowing them to leap out of bed, but that then leads to the classic mid-afternoon slump involving fatigue and sugar cravings at about 3p.m. (a classic sign of waning cortisol production). Sometimes generally low levels can be seen throughout the day; in which case even getting out of bed can literally become a drag (and this would characterise the adrenal exhaustion phase). The sleep hormone melatonin is the primary hormone in the body that opposes cortisol production, which is incredibly relevant to those that are still in an overproductive state, as they will need to reduce their excessive cortisol production (before the reserve starts to 'run dry') by getting precious sleep. Something to consider for shift workers and those with difficulties sleeping.

This test can therefore assist in addressing overproduction of cortisol before it leads to underproduction, and also assists in demonstrating exactly when support and attention to balance is most required throughout the day. We could all do with a little warning before discomfort and incapacitation dictates the solution.

—Warren Maginn, functional clinical nutritionist

Adrenaline and noradrenaline

Adrenaline and noradrenaline are both released by the adrenal glands into the bloodstream in response to stress (noradrenaline is also a neurotransmitter). Together, along with cortisol, these hormones increase your breathing and heart rate, dilate your pupils and restrict blood flow to your kidneys and gastrointestinal tract. They also dilate blood vessels that supply organs involved in exercise (such as your muscles and your heart, so you can run from the bear) and release glucose from the liver. In addition, all non-essential functioning (essential being what is needed to fight or run from the bear) grinds to a halt. So things like your digestion and immune defences slow right down or even stop.

Stopping or even slowing down digestion has huge ramifications on your health. You cannot digest and assimilate the vitamins and nutrients you need from your food if you are chronically stressed, and this can lead to nutritional deficiencies. Your gastrointestinal tract moves by way of something called peristalsis (how a little caterpillar moves) and stopping this movement can lead to things such as constipation. Remember, you will not be digesting food or wanting to poo if you are running from a bear!

Stress also affects your mood, memory, concentration, drive and libido, and can make you crave sweet or fatty foods. It really is one of those sneaky little things that has big knock-on effects in other parts of your life you may not have recognised.

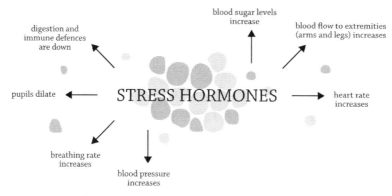

What happens when you are preparing to run from a bear!

As I have mentioned before, this process is supposed to happen for a short period of time—while you're running from or fighting that bear. There is not meant to be a bear in front of you ALL THE TIME. If exposed to stress all the time, your adrenal glands get depleted and your health goes downhill.

Chronic stress is associated with weight gain, obesity, heart disease, infertility, high blood pressure, chronic fatigue syndrome, allergies, metabolic syndrome (syndrome X), diabetes, persistent colds and leaky-gut syndrome—to name just a few.

You need to take a look at all the stressors in your life to see which ones you can modify and which ones you have to live with (but you may be able to change your response to them), in order to reduce your stress to help your health.

In Chapter 15 I'll cover some little tricks and ways of reducing your stress, so if you are feeling all inspired and want to start now, flick over to Chapter 15 (unless it is past 10p.m. at night, and if that is the case, go to bed!).

CHAPTER 6

Gut microflora and your health

I am a nutritionist, so you would be right in thinking that I love food! Possibly you would think that I believe that good health starts with eating good food, right? Wrong. It actually starts in the GUT! This is one thing that was drummed into me during my studies and I must say it is the best thing I have ever learned. If you want to gain and maintain good health—it all has to start in your gut. You can put the best organic/biodynamic/grass-fed anything in your mouth but unless you digest it properly and you have good balanced gut flora, it is all going to waste and can even cause you more harm than good.

Good health really does start within the gut, but I find that it is one of the most overlooked aspects of people's health. Good gut health is paramount to your wellbeing, and I don't just mean physically. Good or bad gut health has implications in all areas of your health, including your psychological wellbeing—yes, the bugs can influence whether or not you are happy or sad!

The gut is the epicentre of our immune system. It is the main defensive barrier that your body has to keep the bad guys out. Anything that you eat and drink has the potential to be swarming with bad bugs, and while still in your small intestine it is technically still 'outside' your body. This is until it passes through the lining of your intestine and into the bloodstream. While it is still on the 'outer', you're still safe from any hidden nasties hanging about in what you just ate. Did you know that the number of bacteria colonising the mucosal and skin surfaces on the body exceeds the number of actual cells forming the human body? The human gut alone contains on average 40,000 bacterial species, 9 million unique bacterial genes and 100 trillion microbial cells. Our human genes are massively outnumbered by these bacterial genes and this enormous diversity of bacteria in the gut has been likened to the diversity of a rainforest. This is actually a great analogy for looking at what goes on in our gut. It is a diverse, interconnected, delicate ecosystem, where things need to be kept in balance in order to maintain harmony (good health).

These commensal bacteria (the normally harmless bacteria that co-exist within us), under specific conditions, can also pose some problems when they are able to overrun our protective responses and exert pathological effects. In much the same way that external environmental threats (invading pathogens) can do the same. This is when our 'rainforest' starts to get unbalanced and the 'deforestation' starts.

Disturbances of this delicate balance, due to external or internal factors, are known to result in many inflammatory and immunological conditions, which can then have knock-on effects.

> Good health really does start within the gut but it is one of the most overlooked aspects of people's health.

Most of us know that there are opposing armies of bacteria running around in our gut. Some of them are friendlies', others are not so friendly (more like the enemy faction)! The good guys work with the mucus layer and the immune barrier in the gut. The mucus layer is secreted by goblet cells, which are cells that secrete mucin. When mucin dissolves in water, it forms mucus. The immune barrier consists of secretory IgA and immune cells such as macrophages or natural killer cells (how cool do those guys sound?) and neutrophils. These guys all work together, supporting our gut health and immune function.

Commensal bacteria are known to provide an excellent hurdle against the excessive colonisation of the gut by pathogenic bacteria by making sure they have enough numbers to 'crowd out' the bad guys. They even communicate directly with your intestinal tissue, recognising bacteria and their toxic products.

These good bugs should be considered an integral component of our immune function. Research is showing us more and more that there are detrimental health implications when we come under enemy fire from the bad bacteria in the gut and they start to gain ground and multiply. So, what are some of the common ways that the bad guys gain the upper ground?

Antibiotics

- Yes, antibiotics have their place in medicine, but we also now know that they should not be overused. Antibiotic use has been shown to have the most common and significant impact on gut microflora. How badly antibiotics affect your gut bacteria will depend on the length of the course, dosage, rate of intestinal absorption and the spectrum of activity (the sorts of bacteria it targets).

- Recent epidemiological research suggests that a single course of antibiotics may have an effect on gut microflora for up to sixteen months after use, compared to individuals who had not taken any antibiotics during the same period of time.

- Antibiotic use can also encourage the overgrowth of opportunistic, already present organisms such as *Clostridium difficile.*

Stress (both physical and psychological)

- It has been theorised that stress-induced changes in gut responses, such as inhibition of gastric acid release and altered gut motility (which are all related to your 'fight or flight' stress response), result in an intestinal environment that is less beneficial to the survival and replication of particular strains of good bacteria. This reduction in survival and replication results in increased numbers of potentially pathogenic bacteria.

- Exercise causes cortisol to be released and a stress response occurs—this is why if you are having issues with gut health, strenuous exercise might not be the best thing for you.

- The gut also plays host to large numbers of neuroendocrine hormones such as serotonin and noradrenaline (norepinephrine). Exposure to stress leads to sudden and sometimes sustained increases in noradrenaline, which may result in increased growth of the bad guys in your gut (not a good thing!).

Diet

- A diet high in simple sugars and refined carbohydrates slows down bowel transit times and increases bacterial fermentation activity. This can lead to increased exposure to potentially toxic bowel contents. It has also been observed that large amounts of ingested sugar lead to a high output of bile acids. Bile acids are actually utilised by some particular gut bugs as food, hence they get an opportunistic advantage over other bug groups and an imbalance in the 'rainforest' develops.

- Preservatives and additives, such as sulphates and sulphites, have also been shown to increase the growth of potentially bad bacteria in the gut.

- Lactose intolerance can cause an overgrowth of bad bacteria in the gut, leading to leaky-gut syndrome.

- Diets with excess protein consumption or maldigestion of protein, due to the fact that undigested protein is fermented by the microflora in the colon, lead to excess ammonia production.

- The consumption of alcohol has been shown to adversely impact the tight gap junctions in the intestine, thus promoting leaky gut. This continual assault on the gut barrier puts the gut cells more at risk of infection and the potential for opportunistic bacteria to overdevelop.

These are not the ONLY ways the bad guys can get the upper hand, but they tend to be some of the most common.

Good gut health really does start from the moment you are born, and in saying this, *how* you are born plays a big part.

Babies develop their commensal bacteria from a number of ways: from liquid ingested during passage through the birth canal; from breastfeeding (babies who are bottle-fed may have bacteria ten times lower than that of babies who are breast-fed, and babies who are born via caesarean section have a much slower development of good bacteria). All of this is crucial to the baby developing a healthy immune system for their future. A review of several studies by Koplin et al. found that caesarean-section babies and bottle-fed babies have a higher risk of developing asthma, allergies and other immune-regulated conditions later in life. This also highlights the reason why pregnant and breastfeeding mums need to have tip-top bugs themselves, to pass on to their little ones. In Chapter 13 I will cover what you can do to give your baby the best start for good gut health.

So, now you know how important it is to maintain good bugs, but they are only one part of the good-gut equation. Good gut health is a combination of good (commensal) bacteria, healthy appropriate defence responses (immunity) and good functioning of the mucosal barrier.

Intestinal permeability, or leaky gut, is a term that has been used in naturopathic medicine for years, but it is still generally not recognised by mainstream medicine. The gut not only acts as a place for digestion and the absorption of nutrients, but also as a barrier between the 'inside' and 'outside' environments. You see, while food and drink are in your small intestine, they are still technically on the 'outer'. They have not yet passed through into the bloodstream. Intestinal permeability is when your intestinal wall starts to let things through into your body that it should not, causing all sorts of mayhem!

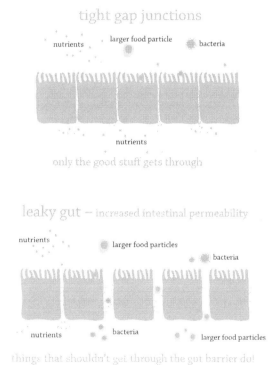

The intestinal wall, or barrier, is bombarded with a huge amount of the bad guys it is trying to keep out, from large portions of undigested food to bacteria and invading viruses. This barrier is a lining with many tight, intact junctions that, when functioning properly, only lets through small broken-down nutrients that your body recognises into the bloodstream.

When you consume foods that you are not able to digest properly, or when your body is not functioning properly due to a host of different reasons such as stress, malnutrition, infection or altered bacteria, food particles that are not broken down sufficiently manage to pass through a 'loose' or weakened lining and on into the bloodstream. The body tags these larger particles as being foreign and sets in motion components of the immune system to attack these foreign particles, the same way it would if there were an actual bacteria or virus attacking the body. The end-product of all this is chronic inflammation and oxidative damage (not a good thing at all!).

Intestinal permeability can be affected by many things, and like so many adverse health conditions in the modern world, it is generally not just one thing, but the accumulative effects of many constant little things. The over consumption of refined foods, grains, legumes, pasteurised dairy or even foods that an individual has an allergy to, malnutrition, medications such as antibiotics, non-steroidal anti-inflammatory drugs (NSAIDs) and antacids, stress and alcohol can all affect intestinal permeability. Did you know that malnutrition is very common in the modern world? Even in First World countries due to our calorie-dense, nutrient-deficient 'fast food'. These are just some of the ways you can cause too much stress on your intestinal barrier and end up with a leaky gut.

What are the main mechanisms driving disturbances to gut integrity and function?

The balance of bacteria living within our digestive system is becoming increasingly acknowledged in the scientific literature as one of the primary determinants of not only our gut and digestive function, but also our immune and nervous system function. So, the relevance of microflora to overall health is perhaps underappreciated and all too commonly overlooked simply for no other reason than a lack of understanding on how to assess it and address it (such as via a Comprehensive Stool Analysis (CSA) and the judicious use of anti-microbial agents and prebiotic/probiotic supplementation).

But before we can make best use of flora assessments and probiotic regimes, we need to ensure the integrity of the gut lining in the first place, to 'house' the native flora effectively and reduce other inflammatory issues such as food allergens crossing the compromised gut membrane and emerging within the bloodstream to drive rampant inflammation in multiple tissues around the body.

The clinical test we use to assess gut lining permeability is the Intestinal Permeability (IP) Test, which involves administering a simple sugar solution containing lactulose (a large molecule of two sugar units) and mannitol (a small simple sugar that should easily transport through the gut cells) before collecting the urine for a six-hour period. This allows us to determine how 'leaky' the gut is by seeing how much lactulose was absorbed (between the cells), compared with how well it absorbs what it should (mannitol absorption indicates the gut cell's ability to effectively absorb basic nutrients such as amino acids and simple carbohydrates in the course of normal digestion). A problematic scenario would be too much 'leaking' (high lactulose absorption) and not enough 'absorbing' (low mannitol absorption) suggesting 'nutrient malabsorption' and 'leaky gut', that tends to come from a blunting of the absorptive microvilli surfaces of the digestive tract, as a result of damage, malnutrition and inflammation.

Sufficient absorptive capacity of select nutrients is required to nourish the body and ultimately provide it with enough resources to maintain the health and integrity of connective tissue. Therefore, the consequences of intestinal permeability being brought about by gut inflammation (from a high allergenic load or pathogenic flora overgrowth) and/or a depleting supply of nutrients to maintain its integrity, causes a vicious circle that, to be broken, requires Removal of the injurious factors, Repair of the damaged membrane, Replenishment of the nutrients deficiencies and the Reinoculation of the digestive system with the beneficial microflora that will ultimately maintain and optimise the health of the tissue going forward. (These principles constitute a version of the '4 Rs' described within classic naturopathic medicine that has long regarded the gut as the centre of health and disease in the body.)

It should perhaps also be noted how stress undermines the ability to even begin this process (of maintaining a healthy gut lining), by switching the nervous system into 'sympathetic dominance' which basically prioritises all body functions to those of IMMEDIATE response/reaction to external threats or requirements, and therefore leaves the digestive system 'high and dry' as a secondary priority to our immediate survival. We have all heard of the saying 'you look like you've seen a ghost' when the blood has rushed from our face when under stress. Well, the same applies to the gut. When we are shocked, tense, afraid, uneasy etc. our gut also drains of blood flow, deviating those crucial resources to wherever the body feels is the more appropriate distribution of resources at that moment. However, if relaxation or the resolution of that pressure never comes, and we remain in an ongoing state of tension (very common within modern lifestyles), the gut tissue never gets the 'air time' it needs to recover, regenerate and serve as our most primary interface with the outside world and therefore to successfully act as our primary site of defence and to obtain the essential (repair) nutrients we need. Just another mechanism by which stress (especially the insidious and ongoing kind) can undermine our overall health, wellbeing and personal potential on a VERY core level.

—Warren Maginn, functional clinical nutritionist

Some of the conditions commonly associated with poor gut health and chronic inflammation are:

- Allergies

- Coeliac disease

- Crohn's disease

- Inflammatory bowel disease (IBD)

- Irritable bowel syndrome (IBS)

- Eczema and psoriasis, and

- Ulcerative colitis.

Some other conditions that you may not know are associated with gut health and chronic inflammation include:

- Depression and mood disorders

- Female reproductive issues—hormonal imbalances, oestrogen dominance, polycystic ovary syndrome (PCOS), infertility, premenstrual syndrome (PMS)

- Atherosclerosis

- Periodontal disease

- Obesity and diabetes, and

- Colon cancer.

The more we continue to study, the more we realise how little we know about our gut ecology and how it influences our health and wellbeing. One thing we do know for sure is that if we want to remain in good health and lead a happy and healthy life, even as we age, good gut health is imperative. In Chapter 13, I will cover how to repair your gut health and how to keep your good bugs happy!

CHAPTER 7

Inflammation—the hidden culprit

We are what we eat! How many times have you heard that saying over the years? Well, it's true and what you eat has huge ramifications on your body with regards to your immunity and inflammation.

You might have figured out already from the previous chapters that I love to harp on about inflammation and, more importantly, systemic or chronic inflammation. Why? Because I believe that controlling the inflammatory pathways in your body is one of the MOST IMPORTANT ways you can practise preventative medicine to keep yourself healthy and well—not only now, but as you continue to grow older.

Much like every other process in the body, inflammation is a necessary process and serves a purpose, but it is when things get out of whack that inflammation becomes a big issue for you and your health.

Inflammation is a natural defence mechanism by your body firstly, to protect an injured site and then, ultimately, to help it to heal. Think of a cut, an insect bite, a broken bone or some sort of trauma—you get the picture. It is actually your immune system that sets off this chain of events that causes the inflammation, through the release of chemical mediators (little messengers). These little messengers are responsible for affecting the blood vessels, nerves and tissue fluid in the local area, causing the symptoms associated with inflammation, such as swelling, blood clotting, pain and fever, which are the beginnings of the healing process.

The immune system

Your immune system is your caped crusader—the defender of your universe (your body) and when he is working his normal nine-to-five job, he does it well. He knows who should be in your body and who shouldn't. Remember in Chapter 6 when we were talking about leaky gut? Well, when undigested particles of food are continually getting through a leaky intestinal wall lining, your caped crusader is working overtime! While he is busy always fighting off the bad guys, the rest of your body has limited defences, leading to increased infections and opportunistic bugs running rampant elsewhere. Not only that, he is tired, so he is only fighting at about 20 per cent of his capacity and not really concentrating on who he is actually fighting. He may end up fighting some of the good guys, and this is when you potentially start to develop new food allergies, or worse, when you develop autoimmune disorders (where your caped crusader thinks your own cells are the bad guys).

Acute inflammation versus chronic inflammation

Acute inflammation is exactly as it sounds—it generally has a rapid onset and is fairly short in duration (although you can have a delayed onset and more prolonged acute inflammation, e.g. sunburn). It flares up quickly, is usually localised to the area that has sustained the injury or illness and disappears when the healing job is done. All good.

Chronic inflammation develops when the cause of the inflammation has not been completely eradicated or the irritation is ongoing. This is not a good place to be. Your caped crusader is feeling endlessly under attack and you permanently have an immune system running below par.

Now, how do omega-6s fit in to this chronic inflammatory situation? Well, you know how we were talking about the chemical messengers that get released during the immune response? They are synthesised (made) from arachidonic acid—the pro-inflammatory omega-6. So, if you have loads and loads of omega-6 in your body, you will always be in a pro-inflammatory state. And it is a fairly safe bet these days to say that the average person, consuming an average Western-style diet, will have some level of inflammation going on in their system. Most of them will have A LOT of inflammation!

Chronic inflammation is linked to many lifestyle conditions such as an increased risk of cardiovascular disease, diabetes, insulin resistance, obesity, arthritis, joint pain, asthma, allergies, metabolic syndrome (syndrome X), fibromyalgia, polycystic ovary syndrome (PCOS), migraines, high blood pressure, diverticulitis, eczema and much, much more.

The thing is, a lot of this inflammation can go unnoticed, get written off as 'well, that's just me' or it may continue to fly under the radar undetected. That does not mean it is a healthy way to live and it can still lead to some serious health consequences down the track.

I have heard countless times from clients with inflammatory conditions, such as irritable bowel syndrome, eczema or arthritis, that it is 'just me' and they think they are destined to live with the condition when, more often than not, they simply do not have to. Many of these inflammatory conditions can diminish significantly or, better yet, disappear altogether, through adopting an anti-inflammatory diet and doing some gut repair.

The scary thing is most people just treat the issue symptomatically with anti-inflammatory drugs, such as aspirin or ibuprofen. These generally work by blocking some part of the 'chain of events' that the immune system has set off. A system that the body has in place for a reason—to warn you something is not right and it is trying to protect itself. Not only do these drugs have a host of side effects, but you are also not fixing the root of the problem! The cause of the inflammation is still there. The inflammation is still there. It is just that you can't 'hear' the signal anymore, whether that be a headache, itchy skin or high blood pressure. People just want the headache to be gone, the itchy skin to disappear or the high blood pressure to go away. I get that—I don't want a headache either! But recognise it for what it is: *a symptom of an underlying cause.*

As a holistic practitioner I was taught to always go looking for the underlying cause of a problem, not just treat it symptomatically. And that is what I want you to do. Know that nearly all chronic inflammatory conditions are associated with poor gut health. If you reduce your inflammation and heal your gut, you will be a lot closer to living a healthy, pain-free, medication-free life.

Reducing inflammation

Inflammation can be the cumulative effect of many little factors. To work out the cause of any inflammation, try the following steps.

- Find out if you have any food intolerances.

- Remove all pro-inflammatory foods from your diet (refer to chapters 2 and 3).

- Heal your gut and keep your good bugs happy (refer to Chapter 13).

- Reduce your stress (have you taken the quick stress quiz in Chapter 5?).

- Use food as medicine (refer to Chapter 11).

- Get enough sleep (your body does its best healing when you are asleep).

- Normalise your weight (the ideal weight at which your body functions optimally).

- If you are sick or injured, REST!

How do you know if you have chronic inflammation?

Many people do not recognise the potential symptoms of chronic inflammation in their body, and at times the inflammation can go unnoticed. My best advice would be to see a natural health practitioner or an integrative doctor. They will take an in-depth look at your health history and can order any tests (if necessary) to assess the inflammatory markers in your body.

What are some of the long-term consequences of ongoing chronic inflammation?

One of the main results of unchecked inflammation is ... well ... more inflammation. (There is a tendency for inflammation to cause a self-perpetuating cycle of further inflammation if a number of self-regulation systems don't bring a stop to it.)

The reason for this is that while inflammation is your body's natural response to threat or injury, and does initiate much of the initial processes of healing, there is almost always some 'collateral damage' that the body accepts in the course of dealing with whatever it feels to be a priority. An example of this would be the tendency for various mediators of inflammation to cause an increase in the permeability of tissues and blood vessels to allow white blood cells (such as neutrophils) to pass through these previously intact barriers, in order to access regions of tissue under threat or requiring clean up and repair.

The body also has some key 'self-resolution' systems that it employs to resolve inflammation, such as the differentiation of T Lymphocytes (white blood cells) from Th1 and Th2 'helper cells' (that support inflammatory processes around the body) to become 'Treg' (regulator) and 'Th3' cells that down-regulate inflammation in the body by suppressing key inflammatory molecules like 'tumour necrosis factor alpha' (TNF-a) via 'transforming growth factor beta' (TGF-b) (one of the most significant anti-inflammatory compounds produced in the body—actually within the gut to be specific, in response to signals from 'friendly' gut bacteria) in the assumption that the threat has surely been addressed and less reactivity is now the most appropriate mode for the immune system to take (in order to preserve resources for future threats, and minimise any further damage to 'self' tissues), since the default response of the immune system must always be 'tolerance' the vast majority of the time, if we are to survive very long.

Some of the most deleterious elements that encourage inflammation within the body are:

1. Allergies: Sensitivity reactions to foods and environmental components.

2. Dysbiosis: The presence of bacterial infections and the absence of 'friendly' gut bacteria supported by a healthy digestive system and a whole-food diet.

3. Thoughts: There is even some evidence to suggest that negative, stressful thoughts or even the mere recollection of negative memories can increase inflammatory activity within the body.

4. Tissue fats: The balance of omega-6 and omega-3 in our tissues, which if stacked too highly in favour of omega-6 will practically dictate that even the mildest of cellular responses must be inflammatory (regardless of the stimuli).

So, some of the most profound strategies we can employ to resolve long-term inflammation, and bring about a reduction/resolution to the ongoing damage constantly requiring repair, are:

• Fish oil supplements: Rectify the tissue balance of omega-6 to omega-3 (to a ratio of no more than 5:1 using Red Blood Cell Lipid testing to find out how to determine this). Use extremely high quality fish oil supplements that have been shown to have the lowest detectable levels of metal and chemical toxin residues as well as the lowest oxidation rates and are in the most stable and absorbable 'triglyceride' form (closest to simply eating a piece of fish) and contain achievable concentrations of both EPA and DHA fatty acids in the order of grams per daily dose/s.

• Probiotics: Rectifying any dysbiosis (the absence of various essential gut flora and the presence of potential parasites and pathogens) so that ample beneficial flora can enhance TNF-a. Note: Bifido species constitute a large portion of healthy colonic flora and so products that support their numbers specifically would perhaps be most prudent (multiple billions of live organisms are required to derive any therapeutic effect and so a cheap way of exceeding the numbers found in even the highest quality probiotic supplements is to culture foods with those probiotic strains and maximise their numbers and activity before ingestion that way).

• Relaxation: Addressing stress and feeling that ultimately our environment is safe and 'all is essentially well' in our lives (because if we don't believe it in our minds, nor will our immune cells—and we are therefore likely to be more 'reactionary' in both body and mind). Who knew having a short fuse made you more likely to have reason to have a short fuse?

Break any of these obstructive cycles and you can start optimising and maintaining a more favourable equilibrium for your long-term health and happiness today. One that says, 'I belong here, and I am at peace with my environment'—something that all humans were born with the potential for.

—Warren Maginn, functional clinical nutritionist

CHAPTER 8

What is Paleo?

So, what is Paleo? 'Paleo' is short for Paleolithic—referring to the Paleolithic era of human history. The Paleo diet has gained huge popularity and momentum in the past few years, with the words 'Paleo diet' ranked up there on Google Trends as one of the hottest searches. This 'Paleo' approach to eating is also sometimes referred to in the media as: the primal diet, real-food diet, whole-food diet, caveman diet, the Grok diet, hunter–gatherer diet, ancestral diet, traditional-foods diet, Stone Age diet and the grain-free, sugar-free and dairy-free diet.

Paleo is about eating nutrient-dense foods that consist mostly of meats, vegetables, fruit, nuts and seeds, while eliminating or reducing foods that are problematic for you. I believe that it should also include a strong emphasis on *living* a life that is also conducive to bettering your health. This means getting adequate sleep, making sure you exercise, having plenty of social interactions (and no, Facebook does not count!) and reconnecting with nature. It is about looking at our evolutionary biology and our ancestors and seeing where we have made some wrong turns with our food choices (and lifestyle) and consequently how these have negatively impacted our health.

The Paleo approach is not about replicating the caveman way of life. We actually do not know exactly what was eaten back then! It is about looking at our biology and figuring out what is the most nutrient-dense food we can eat to nourish our body, prevent disease and lead a healthy life. This means making choices to not consume highly processed foods, foods high in anti-nutrients and where possible, to buy local, seasonal and sustainable foods.

Where things get murky is the fact that a good diet for me may not be a good diet for you. Some foods may be extremely healthy, but a particular individual eating that food might actually become sick or feel unwell. Does that mean that person should continue to eat that food just because it is deemed 'healthy'? No. Therefore, my version of Paleo is not your version of Paleo and vice versa. Nor should it be! We are all individuals and our diet should reflect this. This is where I follow (and treat my clients with) a Paleo template, coupled with a naturopathic point of view. The Naturopathic Medicine principles that I adhere to are the following:

1. First, do no harm.

2. Nature has healing powers.

3. Identify and treat the cause.

4. Treat the whole person.

5. The physician is a teacher.

6.   Prevention is the best cure.

7.   Establish health and wellness.

What does this all mean? Well, it means that it is my job to share this health information with you. It means that we need to have nature involved in our lives again—to get out and put our feet in the grass! It means that there is no quick fix and you must always be looking for the root cause of an issue, not just skim across the top and treat the superficial symptoms. It also means that you must be invested in your own health and practise preventative medicine. Get yourself well and actively keep yourself well. It doesn't happen by just taking a pill. There is some work involved and you are the only one who can do it. You can't always put your health in the hands of others—take ownership!

I believe that the study of nutrition is still in its infant stages and what we know and think is correct today may be different to what we know and think is correct in the future. So let's not pretend that we know everything! The key is to try to continually be open to new ideas and information, consume real food, don't sweat the small stuff and get out in nature. Live a fulfilling life and strive to be the healthiest version (in both mind and body) of OURSELVES we can be.

How do you make Paleo work for you?

The first thing you need to ask yourself is why you have decided to give Paleo a go. Write it down and explore the reasons. I ask you to do this because I want you to acknowledge if you are truly only doing this for weight loss. Don't get me wrong, I am all for everyone maintaining a healthy weight, but if you are ONLY doing this to 'get a bikini body', you are missing the point. I want you to write down why you want to do this, then think about it and really ask yourself why.

Yes, your weight will balance out by doing Paleo, but many, many people out there have tried Paleo for weight loss and have failed miserably. Why? Because they have only looked at the symptom (weight gain) rather than the root cause (the real underlying issue) for their weight gain. Maybe they have hormonal imbalances. This prevents a lot of people from losing weight, even if they are eating perfect Paleo food. Maybe they have poor gut health or digestive issues. Maybe they have huge amounts of stress in their life which they are not acknowledging. As you know from the previous chapters, this will also prevent you from losing weight. Maybe they have self-esteem issues, bad relationships with food, are not getting enough sleep, or are exercising too much—the list goes on and on. You must take care of these issues as well as change the way you eat. You need to look after the WHOLE you. This may mean that you need to book an appointment to see a counsellor or a therapist, possibly not something you thought you would be considering by 'going Paleo'. But trust me, if you really want to be happy and healthy, you need to look after ALL of you!

I want you to try Paleo is so you can be the healthiest and happiest version of yourself—in all aspects of your life.

I want you to try Paleo so you can be the healthiest and happiest version of yourself—in all aspects of your life, not just from a weight perspective. So please, let's 'treat the whole person' and do this for the right reasons. I am more excited for you to show me the good blood results you will get, rather than the weight-loss figures. I am more excited for you to tell me you are excited by life again and have reduced your stress levels. That you are sleeping well and have reduced your inflammation. I am more excited that you will tell me that you have found a love for good food and you are using 'food as medicine' to stay well. Trust me, do it for these reasons—the right reasons—and the weight will take care of itself.

Many people after being Paleo for some time end up doing an 80/20 version of a Paleo way of eating. This means they eat Paleo foods 80 per cent of the time and non-Paleo foods 20 per cent of the time. I am not going to tell you that 80/20 is right or 90/10 is right or even that you must be 100 per cent Paleo all of the time. This is for you to figure out for yourself. But I would like you to keep this quote in mind:

> *Do not be so rigid or self-righteous about your diet as to annoy anyone. A bad relationship is more poisonous than one of Grandma's sugar cookies.*

—Paul Pitchford, author of *Healing with Whole Foods*

Life is meant for living and to be enjoyed! I don't want you causing yourself or your family and friends huge amounts of stress over what to eat. What is the point of that? You know by now how damaging stress can be for you. Yes, be true to yourself and the way you eat, but don't stress about the small stuff. Eating out with friends or enjoying Christmas dinner with your family is about cherishing the company, celebrating and enjoying the experience. Don't stress about what you ate or drank. You can still make 'healthier' choices during these events, but like my husband says, 'Unless you are allergic to cookies, eating one is not going to make you explode!' So, when it comes time for you to go to one of these events, take a 'Paleo leave-pass' and have a good time—nutritionist's orders!

I can hear you asking: *Well, WHAT exactly am I meant to be eating then?* Meats, vegetables, fruit, nuts and seeds, while eliminating or reducing problematic foods, of course! Let's take a look at what this may look like. Opposite are some lists that I have compiled of what you would generally find in my kitchen. These are by no means the only foods available, but they will give you a great starting point.

General Paleo foods

VEGETABLES

Asian greens (bok choy, choy sum, pak choy)

Artichoke

Asparagus

Avocado

Bamboo shoots

Beetroot (beets)

Broccoli (broccolini)

Brussels sprouts

Cabbage

Capsicum (peppers)

Carrot

Cauliflower

Celeriac

Celery

Cucumber

Daikon

Eggplant (aubergine)

Endive (chicory)

Fennel

Green beans

Horseradish

Jerusalem artichoke

Jicama

Kale

Kohlrabi

Leek

Lettuce

Mushrooms

Okra

Olives

Onions

Parsnips

Potatoes

Pumpkins

Radishes

Sea vegetables (dulse, kombu, wakame, nori and kelp)

Shallots

Silverbeet (chard)

Snow peas (mangetout)

Spinach

Spring onions (scallions)

Squash

Sugar snap peas

Swede (rutabaga)

Sweet potato (kumara)

Taro

Tomatoes

Turnips

Yams

Zucchini (courgette)

Zucchini flower

FRUITS

Apples

Apricots

Bananas

Blackberries

Blood oranges

Blueberries

Boysenberries

Cherries

Cranberries

Cumquats

Currants

Custard apples

Dragon fruit

Figs

Gooseberries

Grapefruit

Grapes

Guava

Honeydew melon

Kiwi fruit

Lemons

Limes

Loganberries

Loquats

Lychees

Mandarins

Mangoes

Mangosteens

Medjool dates

Mulberries

Nashi pears

Naval oranges

Nectarines

Papaya (pawpaw)

Passionfruit

Peaches

Pears

Persimmons

Pineapple

Plums

Pomegranates

Quinces

Rambutan

Raspberries

Rhubarb

Rockmelon (cantaloupe)

Star fruit

Strawberries

Tamarillo

Tangelo

Valencia oranges

Watermelon

MEATS AND EGGS

Beef

Chicken

Duck

Eggs

Goat

Goose

Kangaroo

Lamb

Lobster

Mackerel

Morton Bay bugs

Mussels

Mutton

Oysters

Pork

Prawns

Quail

Rabbit

Salmon

Sardines

Scallops

Shrimp

Snapper

Squab

Trout

Tuna

Turkey

Veal

Venison

Yabbies

NUTS AND SEEDS

Almonds

Brazil nuts

Chia seeds

Coconut

Hazelnuts

Macadamia nuts

Pecans

Pine nuts

Pistachios

Pumpkin seeds (pepitas)

Sesame seeds

Sunflower seeds

Walnuts

FATS AND OILS

Avocado oil

Butter (pastured)

Coconut oil

Duck fat

Ghee

Macadamia oil

Olive oil

Sesame oil

HERBS AND SPICES

Aniseed

Annatto

Basil

Bay leaf

Caraway

Cardamom

Cayenne pepper

Chilli

Chives

Cinnamon

Cloves

Coriander (cilantro)

Cumin

Dill

Fennel

Fenugreek

Five spice

Galangal

Garlic

Garam masala

Ginger

Kaffir lime leaves (makrut)

Lavender

Lemongrass

Lemon myrtle

Marjoram

Mint

Mountain pepper

Mustard

Nutmeg

Oregano

Paprika

Parsley

Peppercorn (white and black)

Peppermint

Rosemary

Saffron

Salt (pink Himalayan)

Sawtooth coriander

Star anise

Tarragon

Thai basil

Thyme

Turmeric

Vanilla

LIQUIDS/DRINKS

Almond milk

Bone broth

Cashew milk

Coconut milk

Coconut water

Herbal tea

Kombucha

Organic coffee

Soda water

Tea (black and green)

Water

SWEETENERS (OCCASIONAL USE)

Coconut sugar

Fruit juice and fruit purée

Honey (raw)

Maple syrup (pure)

Medjool dates

Palm sugar

Stevia

OTHER PANTRY AND FRIDGE ITEMS

Almond meal

Bee pollen

Cacao butter

Cacao nibs

Cacao powder

Coconut aminos (soy sauce replacement)

Coconut butter

Coconut cream

Coconut flakes

Dark chocolate (+85% cacao)

Dried fruits (sulphur-free)

Fish sauce (gluten free and low sugar)

Kelp noodles

Kimchi

Nut butters (almond, cashew, macadamia)

Sauerkraut

Sun-dried tomatoes

Tahini

Tamarind paste

Tinned salmon and tuna

Tomato paste

Vinegar (apple cider, red wine, balsamic)

Wholegrain mustard

Whole tinned tomatoes

Who ever said eating Paleo was restrictive? Look at the food choices you have at your disposal! Use this as a general starting point of what you will need in your Paleo kitchen, but it is by no means a complete list. And it certainly is not YOUR individualised list! In the next chapter we will talk about creating an individual Paleo plan and what foods can fall into the 'grey foods' category.

CHAPTER 9

Creating an individual Paleo plan

As you can all see from the previous chapter, I am big on treating people as a 'whole'. I believe that it is essential to always find the root cause for health issues, in order for you to be truly happy and healthy. This means that everyone should be treated as an individual and therefore what you eat should also always be tailored to you as an individual.

I cannot tell you exactly HOW much you should eat or exactly WHAT you should eat. That would be me taking your health out of your hands. I want you to gain control of your health again and be pro-active about seeing what actually works for you! I can share my knowledge and give you some general guidelines, but the rest is up to you.

Meal sizes

Generally speaking, you really should not need any more than three meals per day. You don't need any of this 'six meals a day' nonsense, and before you ask—no, eating six meals a day does not speed up your metabolism! We want your normal hormones to do their jobs and, as we saw in Chapter 4, if you are always eating and always releasing insulin, when does glucagon get a chance to do its thing? If you find you need to snack constantly, reassess the size of your meals and make them a little larger (especially breakfast).

The funny thing is, I usually find with my clients that they are often undereating, rather than overeating. So do not be scared to eat! Fill up your plate with all of the good stuff and don't go hungry. Serve a good-sized portion of protein (hand size), fill up the rest of the plate with vegetables and some fruit, and make sure you have some fats and oils in the mix (about 1–2 tablespoons per meal). When you eat real food, your body signals function correctly and when you are hungry, you really are hungry—so eat!

Foods to eat

Sure, there are general 'healthy foods' that I outlined in Chapter 8, but this still does not mean that they are for everyone to eat. My husband can't eat sweet potato. He reacts terribly to it. Does that mean that because it is a nutrient-dense Paleo staple, I am going to keep forcing him to eat it? No, that would just be silly. If you eat a food and it does not sit well with your body, test it out again. If you get the same reaction, don't continue to eat it—even if it is considered a Paleo staple!

Don't just assume, however, that if you react to this food, you will never be able to eat it again. See if your reaction is due to a leaky gut, lack of digestive enzymes or something else that may need to be corrected. Remember to look for the root cause! The reaction to the food may just be the symptom. This is where it also might be wise to seek some professional help to correct any digestive issues you think you might have.

The n=1 food list

I like to call this the n=1 (only one person in the experiment) food list. It is the 'grey foods' list—a list of foods that some people in the Paleo community eat, some do not, or it's one of those foods you just need to find out for yourself if it works well for you and your body. As I have said before, I believe we are still learning about the science of nutrition and therefore we should always be open to finding out new information—and as a result, a list of foods that are suitable to eat is not always so 'black and white'.

For this reason, I think it is essential to experiment with yourself and see how well you tolerate these foods. It is important to note that you should only do this once you have established a clean slate—when you know you have sound gut integrity, you have good digestion and you can recognise the subtleties of your body when having issues with a particular food (see Chapter 16). Also look out for emotional attachments to foods, not just physical reactions (by keeping a DERR diary, see Chapter 17). Do you crave this food at a particular time (say, when you are stressed or before your period if you are female) or do you overeat with this particular food? These are all things you need to note and recognise. Again, engaging the services of a nutritionist to monitor the reintroduction of certain foods might be a good idea.

This list is by no means final. There will always be new things to add as our understanding of nutrition continues to develop. So if you come across anything you want to add, go for it!

THE N=1 FOOD LIST

Full-fat dairy (including goat and sheep milk products)

Some people find they can tolerate goat or sheep dairy.

Full-fat dairy is always a better option than skim or low-fat dairy.

If you have access to raw dairy (if you live on a farm) this is great, as heating dairy can damage the proteins (covered in Chapter 3).

Fat dairy, such as butter and cream, can be handled by most people, even if they cannot tolerate other forms of dairy.

Fermented dairy (kefir and yoghurt)

Fermentation breaks down some of the proteins and sugars that cause people problems.

Make sure the yoghurt is full fat and pot set.

Properly prepared legumes (except soy and peanuts)

Soaking, sprouting, fermenting or cooking beans can reduce the amounts of toxins they contain and make them suitable for people who normally react to them.

Pseudo-grains (quinoa, amaranth and buckwheat)

Some individuals with a healthy gut (no presence of leaky gut) can tolerate these foods.

Proper preparation can also include making sure they are well washed or soaked.

Sprouted beans

Sprouting inactivates most of the toxins, making these safer to eat.

Potato (skin removed) and white rice

These are less problematic when cooked.

Potato and white rice should be eaten in small quantities and only occasionally.

CHAPTER 10

The lowdown on fats, proteins and carbohydrates

Before we get started on this chapter, I would like to make a couple of points. I am a big believer in eating whole foods and trusting your body. Even with my clients, I don't tend to get technical about fat, protein and carbohydrate ratios (aka macronutrients)—but I do think it is important to understand the basics of what these macronutrients offer to your health and wellbeing, and that an eating plan contain all three. Individual foods are not solely made up of just proteins, or just fat, or just carbs—they are a combination of all three (and a whole bunch of other things). There are plenty of books out there where you can delve into the intricate details of macronutrient ratios if you so wish, but I treat people holistically and believe that we need to treat our body in the same manner. In addition, everyone is different and everybody has a different gut function as well as different energy output levels, stress levels, sleep hygiene (how well you sleep), and so on. All of this affects how much you, as an individual, will need of these macronutrients in order to maintain good health.

Rather than focusing on macronutrient ratios, I believe it is far more important to focus on micronutrients (vitamins, minerals and anti-oxidants). How nutrient dense is the food that you are consuming? Does it contain plenty of vitamins, minerals and anti-oxidants per serve? Do you vary your food seasonally so that you are getting a variety of nutrients? All of these things are far more important than the percentage of macronutrients you are consuming. For example, have a look at these two meals below. They contain very similar fat to protein to carbohydrate ratios but do you think one would have more micronutrients per serve than the other and be better for you? You bet one would! (In case you need a hint, the healthy option is not the fish and chips!)

MEAL 1: GRILLED SALMON, MIXED SALAD WITH AVOCADO AND SWEET POTATO

Carbohydrate	25%
Fats	42%
Protein	32%

MEAL 2: FRIED BATTERED WHITE FISH AND CHIPS

Carbohydrate	24%
Fats	45%
Protein	28%

Now let's take a look at some of the micronutrients these meals contain based on a percentage of the daily requirements of a 2000kcal average adult diet.

MEAL 1: GRILLED SALMON, MIXED SALAD WITH AVOCADO AND SWEET POTATO

Vitamin A	493%
Vitamin C	82%
Vitamin B1	44%
Vitamin B2	65%
Vitamin B6	113%
Calcium	12%
Iron	20%
Magnesium	36%
Sodium	9%
Zinc	17%
Omega 3:6	4136mg: 2118mg

MEAL 2: FRIED BATTERED WHITE FISH AND CHIPS

Vitamin A	3%
Vitamin C	16%
Vitamin B1	13%
Vitamin B2	17%
Vitamin B6	28%
Calcium	7%
Iron	10%
Magnesium	23%
Sodium	41%
Zinc	8%
Omega 3:6	953mg: 5138mg

(Source: Nutritiondata.com)

So, what points stand out just from looking at the micronutrient breakdown?

- There are more of your energy-giving B vitamins in Meal 1 and a fantastic ratio of good anti-inflammatory omega-3 fatty acids compared to the high levels of pro-inflammatory omega-6 fatty acids in Meal 2.

- Meal 1 also has good levels of mood-enhancing magnesium and zinc, which is an essential co-factor in hundreds of biochemical pathways in your body.

- Meal 1 has a good boost of vitamins C and A.

- Meal 2 has much lower values of the energy-providing B vitamins.

- Meal 2 is much higher in sodium. Excess sodium in highly processed diets can lead to hypertension (high blood pressure).

My other point is to have a little faith in the wonderful, miraculous thing called your body. Before we knew how to count calories or calculate protein percentages, how on earth did we survive? The really cool thing is your body actually knows how to do this. If you provide it with nutrient-dense, real food, it will take very good care of you and you won't need to count a thing. What you do have to do, though, is strip away all the over processed junk foods from your diet and give your body time to heal, so you can start to listen to the proper signals it is sending you.

So, now that I have that out of my system, let's go over some of the different 'types' of these macronutrients and how they are beneficial to your diet!

Fats

Ah fats, notorious fats! They have been billed as the instigator of bad health and weight gain for years. Eating fat, especially saturated fat, raises our cholesterol levels and gives us heart disease, right? Well, actually no.

Please do me a favour and understand this—eating good healthy fats in your diet will not make you fat and eating saturated fat will not give you cardiovascular disease. Chances are you should be including more fats in your diet than you currently are. They are highly beneficial and also aid in the absorption of fat-soluble vitamins, such as vitamins A, D, E and K.

The whole low-fat (particularly saturated fat) movement started back in the 1950s with a published study that hypothesised that there was a possible relationship between the amount of fat consumed in a diet and the incidence of heart attack. This coupled with the seed-oil production (cottonseed, soybean and corn) of the 1960s and 70s, and cholesterol fear mongering in the 1980s, which has done nothing except cause an exponential increase in the rates of people suffering conditions such as cardiovascular disease, obesity and diabetes.

You only need to go down the aisle of your local supermarket to see the magnitude of 'low fat', 'no fat', 'cholesterol-free' goodies available. All made with love and care to help your health, right? NO! These 'food-like substances' do nothing to enhance your health at all, so stay away from them. There is no substitute for *real* food, as Mother Nature intended—fat and all!

A meta-analysis by Siri-Tarino et al. (a research technique used for combining the findings of independent studies) of 22 studies related to saturated fats and the increased risk of cardiovascular disease found 'that there is no significant evidence for concluding that dietary saturated fat is associated with an increase of CHD (coronary heart disease) or CVD (cardiovascular disease)'. Eating saturated fat is not the problem! But a diet high in saturated fat *and* high in carbohydrates will cause you issues—they are not a good combination. So, are all fats the same?

I don't want to turn this into lipid (fat) learning 101, so I am going to keep things easy. In simple terms we are going to be talking about fatty acids—saturated, monounsaturated, polyunsaturated (including essential fatty acids) and steroids (namely cholesterol).

Fatty acids

A fatty acid contains a carbon chain that is attached to a carboxylic acid. Fatty acids come in different lengths and variations of single or double bonds in the carbon chain and it is these varying lengths that have different effects on the body.

Saturated fats (SAs)

Saturated fats contain only single bonds between carbons. This includes the likes of palmitic acid, found in animal meats and eggs, and lauric acid, which is found in coconut oil. Saturated fats are good to cook with because they have higher smoking points, they are more robust, and you can cook at higher temperatures without doing harm to the oil and your health. They are generally solid at room temperature (except on a hot summer's day!). As we have just learned above, eating saturated fats as part of a healthy diet does not increase your chance of cardiovascular disease and they should be included in your diet.

Monounsaturated fats (MUFAs)

These fats contain only one double bond between carbons and include oleic acid, which is found in olive oil. These guys are very delicate and should not be heated because this damages their anti-oxidant properties. Buy local, good-quality, cold-pressed olive oil (heat processing can damage the oil) and ensure it is in a dark glass bottle so it does not go rancid.

Polyunsaturated fats (PUFAs)

Polyunsaturated fats contain two or more double bonds between carbons. They are also called essential fatty acids (EFAs) as your body cannot make them itself and therefore they need to be obtained through diet. The main players are:

1. Omega-3s: These include docosahexaenoic acid (DHA) and eicosapentaenoic acid (EPA), which are found in oily cold-water fish and algae, and alpha-linolenic acid (ALA) found in flax seeds and chia seeds.

2. Omega-6s: These include arachidonic acid (AA) found in meat and eggs and linoleic acid (LA) found in grains, legumes, vegetable oils, seed oils and nuts.

In general terms (as I covered in Chapter 2) we say that omega-3s are anti-inflammatory and omega-6s are pro-inflammatory. We need them all, but in balance.

Cholesterol

Cholesterol is actually a steroid and is one of the most abundant and important steroids in your body. It is found in the liver, bile salts and skin (where it forms vitamin D) and in your adrenal glands as it is used to make steroid hormones such as aldosterone, cortisol and testosterone. It is also an important component of your cell membranes and your brain and nerve tissue. Cholesterol should not be demonised as the bad guy. With all the cholesterol-lowering drugs around are we really better off? Why is it that about half of the people having heart attacks have cholesterol in 'normal ranges'? It is coming to light that healthy energy-efficient diets rich in fat and cholesterol do not increase total plasma cholesterol. So go on, eat your eggs!

The pathology test commonly used to measure cholesterol levels in the body is not actually 'measuring' cholesterol at all. The test is measuring lipoproteins, the carrier molecules for the cholesterol. Two types of lipoproteins—high-density lipoprotein (HDL) and low-density lipoprotein (LDL)—shuttle cholesterol to and from the liver to different areas of the body to carry out jobs such as cell membrane repair. Both HDL and LDL have important roles in the body and the theory of 'good cholesterol' and 'bad cholesterol' is now being questioned.

Below is a copy of the actual blood tests from a client taken before and then again nine months after following a Paleo template. Look at the improvement in her cholesterol and triglyceride levels. And this is all while eating on average sixteen eggs per week!

	30 JAN 2012	29 SAP 2012
Total Cholesterol (< 5.5)	6.1	5.1
HDL (> 1.1)	1.12	1.8
LDL (< 3.4)	3.9	3
Trig (< 2.0)	2.4	0.7

	30 JAN 2012	29 SAP 2012
CRR (Ave=4.4; Twice Ave=7.0)	5.4	2.8

(Coronary Risk Ratio (CRR) is calculated by dividing the total cholesterol by the HDL level. A higher ratio implies potential higher risk of developing conditions such as coronary artery disease (atherosclerosis).)

Fats that help your health

Omega-3s
These fatty acids in the form of EPA and DHA are found primarily in oily, cold-water fish, such as sardines and anchovies, and in algae and even grass-fed beef. EPA is a powerful anti-inflammatory and improves heart health and circulation. It helps regulate the immune system and is good for joint health. DHA is great for memory and learning, reduces depression and anxiety, and is beneficial for brain and nerve cells. DHA is essential for childhood development and promotes a healthy pregnancy.

Saturated fats
Saturated fats such as coconut oil have antibacterial and antiviral properties and have been shown to be beneficial for people suffering from acne (applied topically and taken internally). They are also beneficial in aiding weight loss, without affecting blood lipid profiles.

Non heat-treated monounsaturated fatty acids (MUFAs)

Olive oil, avocado and nuts have been shown to improve insulin sensitivity, glucose tolerance, reduce cardiovascular disease and even improve sleep. But the secret is DO NOT HEAT THEM and don't buy rancid oils.

Fats that don't help your health

Trans fats

These manmade fats are manufactured by hydrogenating vegetable oils. They are mainly found in over processed foods such as cookies, chips, margarine and baked foods. They are BAD for your health so avoid them at all cost! They disrupt all the good work that the essential fatty acids do and promote inflammation, atherosclerosis, high triglyceride levels and are strongly linked with an increased risk of heart disease.

Heated MUFAs

When oils such as olive oil are heated, they lose a very high percentage of their phenolic components (anti-oxidant properties) and can end up being quiet harmful to your body. Storage is another issue—they need to be kept in dark, sealed bottles or else they can become oxidised and harmful.

Fats that have a foot in both camps!

Arachidonic acid (AA)

This omega-6 gets a bad rap for being a pro-inflammatory agent and yes, that is true, but it is also necessary for the body. It does things like promote inflammation, increase blood clotting, increase pain sensitivity and constrict blood vessels—all critical responses in your body, at particular times. Arachidonic acid is also necessary in pregnancy as it is critical to foetal central nervous system growth and development. It is also involved in cell division and signalling pathways. So you see, it has important *good* jobs it needs to carry out in the body. It is just that with our current lifestyle, we tend to consume *waaaayyy* too much AA—and then we run into issues with chronic inflammation.

Linoleic acid (LA)

Although linoleic acid is found in seeds, nuts, grains and legumes, where we consume it in the largest amount is through vegetable and seed oils, like soybean and canola oil. The United States saw a 5.5-fold increase in canola oil use from 1985–94 and it is the third most consumed oil in the world, with soybean oil leading the way. As we saw in Chapter 2, it is our current balance of omega-6 to omega-3 that is distorted in today's society and it is heavily weighted towards the six—big time! But we still need some omega-6. Having excess omega-6 results in stiff cell membranes, reduced cell communication and limiting nutrients entering the cells. It also means an overproduction of AA and, I'll say it again, CHRONIC INFLAMMATION!

Gamma-linolenic acid (GLA)
Although an omega-6, gamma-linolenic acid is beneficial for health and found primarily in evening primrose oil and borage oil. Research shows that it is beneficial for reducing inflammatory skin conditions, helping with premenstrual syndrome and balancing hormones. When combined with EPA and DHA it is beneficial for children with attention deficit hyperactivity disorder (ADHD) and assists with language and learning difficulties in kids with autism.

So, what can you take away from all this? Have fat with every meal and include a variety of good fats in every meal, including breakfast. Cook with coconut oil and grass-fed butter, have olive oil on your salads and eat oily fish. Your body and your health will thank you for it!

Proteins

Proteins are the building blocks of the body. Large protein molecules are broken down through digestion into single amino acids. These guys are responsible for providing structure in membranes, building cartilage and connective tissue; they act as enzymes, make up components of our immune system and transport oxygen in blood and muscle. They can even be a source of energy for your body.

Protein is one of those macronutrients most people are comfortable with. When I am compiling food plans for my clients, I always get questioned on the fat and carbohydrate levels they should be consuming, but never really protein. Most people (who eat meat) generally eat a reasonable amount of protein. Converting to a Paleo template does not mean you start to eat loads and loads of protein—it is not an 'all meat' diet as some might suggest. Chances are your protein consumption levels will stay close to the same with the exception of one meal: breakfast. The everyday Western-type diet usually kicks off the day with a high-carbohydrate (usually highly processed) meal, something like cereal or toast. Well, I want you to get used to the idea that you will be having some protein and fat with your breakfast. And it is easy to do—it's called eating real food!

Once you have pressed the reset button and devised a weekly meal plan (see chapters 16 and 17), it really is a case of letting your own body signals tell you how much protein you should eat at every meal. A general rule of thumb would be a palm to full-size hand portion per meal.

Good choices of protein are grass-fed meats, as they have a better omega-3 to omega-6 ratio and are raised how nature intended. They are also a good source of conjugated linolenic acid (CLA), which can aid in reducing inflammation and insulin resistance, and assist in weight loss. Wild seafood and pastured poultry and eggs are also great protein choices.

Although some grain-like seeds such as quinoa, or legumes such as beans, are considered reasonable food sources of protein (especially for vegetarians and vegans), they are actually more carbohydrate sources. You are better off getting your protein from animal sources, especially if you want to promote appropriate glucagon responses in your body, which we do!

Carbohydrates

Carbohydrates (carbs for short) seem to cause a whole lot of controversy wherever they go. We are continually being bombarded by today's media with the latest 'research' about how low-carbohydrate diets are bad, sugar is a killer, wholegrains are good or we need to eat complex carbohydrates in order to survive.

I am going to keep things simple and stick to a bit of commonsense. For starters, Paleo is not low carb. It is perhaps lower carb than your average high-carb Western diet, but it does not have to be low carb. Also, everyone is an individual, so I do not want to make statements about the exact amount of carbohydrates a person needs in order to maintain proper health, because for each person it will vary. What I will say is that there are better choices for carbohydrates and there are nutrient-poor choices. There are choices that will enhance your health, and choices that will leave you cranky, hormonally unbalanced and stacking on the weight.

There are people who thrive better on a very low-carb diet (e.g. someone who has epilepsy) and there are people who thrive better on a higher carb diet. I have found in my clinic that most of my clients respond well to being on a moderate carb intake, which can then be tweaked for the individual.

What we need to get out of our heads, though, is that a majority of our meals need to be made up of cereals, breads and pastas. This is just not the case! Your body will flourish when it is allowed to utilise fats as a primary fuel source and it will provide you with balanced, long-lasting energy—no sugar highs and crashes, and no having to eat every hour in order to not get cranky or have your blood sugar levels drop. Carbohydrates are necessary to feed different functions in the body, but your body loves to utilise carbs as a primary fuel source because it is 'quicker and easier'. What is happening in today's society is that far too many carbs are being consumed and the quality of carbs is poor.

Do you remember in Chapter 4 when we were talking about hormones and their role in our body? Well, this is where your quality and quantity of carb intake matters! Remember, insulin is released in response to food coming into your body, but primarily in response to carbs. Well, if you hit your body with a large whack of carbs (sugars), your body has to release a large whack of insulin to mop it up, because too much glucose floating around in the bloodstream is dangerous. If this is happening all day long (because you need to eat every few hours to stop from turning into captain cranky pants) you are always in storage mode.

Glucose gets converted to glycogen, which gets stored in the liver and muscles (to be used as fuel), and once those storage compartments are full, the rest gets converted to fats—in the forms of triglycerides (blood fats) and adipose tissue (body fat). So, can you see the picture forming for Mr Average Joe? He is using carbs as a primary fuel source, so he needs to eat continually for energy, but he is eating too much energy. His glycogen stores are full, because he has a desk job and drives to work and never gets a chance to use up these stores. On the rare occasion he goes to the gym, he still has glucose in his system from his frequent eating, so he burns this as energy and never gets a chance to tap into his fat stores. He ends up packing on excess weight and his triglycerides are on the rise. Not the sort of cycle you want to get stuck in!

It really is as simple as *too many carbs and your body will need to convert them to fat; too few carbs and your body will need to make glucose from proteins* (a process called gluconeogenesis). Neither is an ideal situation to be stuck in for a long period of time. Remember as with most things, your body likes BALANCE.

I do not like to talk in extremes and I try to refrain from such cut-and-dried statements as 'everything is good or bad'. I prefer the terms 'better choices' and 'poorer choices' when talking about carbs.

Better choices for carbohydrates

When adopting a Paleo template, you generally will not be eating grains and so most of your carbs will come in the form of vegetables—some starchy vegetables such as sweet potato, beetroot (beets), pumpkin and parsnips, and some fruits. People on individual plans even eat white potato (gasp!), rice or pseudo-grains such as quinoa. It is about seeing what works for you and making the best choices that will give you a high nutrient intake while not being pro-inflammatory.

So, how much fruit should you eat in a day? You don't have to eat fruit every day, but you can if you want to. It is about finding that 'sweet spot' for you and seeing how many carbs you need to function well. It will depend largely on your output of energy levels and by that I am not just talking about exercise, as convalescing (recovery from illness, healing wounds or operations) will also require more carbohydrates. Also remember that when you are having sufficient protein and fat with your meals and you are using fat as your main fuel source, you do not need to 'snack' constantly and therefore do not need to eat fruit as a quick pick-me-up in-between meals.

I also like to look at the seasons. We have become so far removed from seasonal eating due to the availability of everything in supermarkets all the time. Have you ever noticed that there are a lot more fruits available in summer than in winter? Do we tend to be more active and expend more energy in summer and hibernate more in winter? Yes! And, so it is the same for plants and trees—in the warmer months they produce more fruit than in the colder months. So do something for your health and reduce your carbon footprint at the same time—eat seasonally and buy locally! I have included a seasonal fruit and vegetable guide in Chapter 11.

Poorer choices for carbohydrates

Cereals, pasta and breads—get used to life without them. They are all eaten in excess and are nutritionally poor. Grains also have a whole other element to them in the form of anti-nutrients, which we covered in Chapter 3—all the more reason why they sit in the 'not such a good choice' camp.

Soft drinks, energy drinks, cakes, lollies, chocolates and all those 'junk foods' are also very poor choices. They are calorie dense and nutritionally poor and they do nothing for your health. What about 'sugar free' or 'diet' food and drinks, I hear you ask. *The scientist in a white lab coat cannot out-do nature!* Trust me, these 'franken-foods' are not real foods and they are no good for you. Studies have indicated that consuming these foods actually leads to greater weight gain and can also increase your chances of a heart attack or stroke.

So, how do you make up a nutrient-dense meal? Stay connected with your food. Be real with your food. Don't try to trick yourself that your eating plan needs to be any more difficult than consuming real food, and make sure you have an animal source of protein for every meal, coupled with vegetables and fruit and some natural fats, but don't get too caught up on it. More importantly, know where your food comes from, eat your meals sitting down (do not eat on the run), appreciate the flavours in your food, chew your food well and be grateful for the nutrients it is giving you to help you live a full and healthy life.

What do you feel are some of the most essential nutritional components of a healthy diet?

Well, as mentioned, some of the most essential elements in the diet relate not so much to the *macro* nutrient content, but the *micro* nutrient content. In fact, the ability for plants to properly develop their macronutrients (proteins, fats and carbohydrates) relies primarily on the variety and abundance of minerals present in the soil they are grown in, to act as substrates and cofactors for the formation of those more complex molecules. Animals then simply concentrate these macro- and micronutrients into their tissues (adding some further essential nutrition of their own, via their own metabolism and those of the bacterial flora within their digestive systems, such as in the synthesis of vitamin B12), further illustrating how minerals form the basis to all higher nutrition.

While we can't go past the primacy of minerals (that must first be in our soil, to be in our food, be it plant or animal) to support all further nutrition and our health, we can observe some of the more complex compounds made from them that also fulfil the needs of human nutrition, as we cannot synthesise them ourselves and therefore must acquire them within our diet. Namely the essential fatty acids (fats), essential amino acids (proteins) and essential sugars (carbohydrates)—yes, you read that right, there are essential sugars.

Let's review:

Essential fatty acids: Technically two fatty acids—alpha-linolenic acid (the 'parent' omega-3) and linoleic acid (the 'parent' omega-6)—comprise our essential fatty acids; however, due to the abundance of omega-6 in the modern diet and the inefficiency with which we convert alpha-linolenic acid into its more active downstream derivatives eicosapentaenoic acid (EPA) and docosahexaenoic acid (DHA) (sometimes as low as 0.5 per cent), we also often need to consume abundant amounts of these longer chain omega-3s in the diet. Interestingly, with the exception of algae, these last two fatty acids (EPA and DHA), the most important to modern health, are only obtained through animal foods, most notably fresh fish and their oils.

Essential amino acids: Technically nine amino acids—leucine, isoleucine, valine, histidine, methionine, lysine, threonine, phenylalanine and tryptophan—comprise our essential amino acid building blocks for synthesising all the remaining eleven basic amino acids and the hundreds of thousands of proteins made from them, found within the body. Once again, many of the further eleven amino acids still require external supply due to increased demands put on the human body by modern lifestyles and the inefficient synthesis of these amino acids in certain situations and individuals, particularly within the context of the amount of toxicity we are exposed to in society today. Additionally, the deficiency of even one essential amino acid within the body can hinder the proper utilisation of all the other amino acids. So it is often required that we obtain dietary protein with a fairly complete and balanced profile of amino acids, especially those sufficient in the sulphur-bearing amino acids. Perhaps unsurprisingly, animal proteins tend to be the most complete and balanced sources for meeting these human needs. However, also note that green vegetables have some of the highest percentages of complete protein by dry weight—bringing new meaning to eating your meat and greens.

Essential sugars: Eight sugars have been identified as essential to human health and are gaining increasing focus and research within health science today. These include glucose, galactose, mannose, fucose, xylose, N-acetyl-glucosamine, N-acetyl-galactosamine and N-acetyl-neuraminic acid. They may, in fact, be some of the most crucial determinants of healthy cell function and communication (which for us as an organism as a whole, is as essential as it gets). They do this by providing the essential components to form many of the cell's most primary structures (glycolipids and glycoproteins), particularly on their surface, which allows for their correct differentiation and identification. Their role as 'essential' nutrients is contentious, however, since the first three (glucose, galactose, mannose) are all quite readily available from components of even the most highly processed modern diet and many can be synthesised by the body. Fucose and xylose supply can be readily assured from ample vegetables and to some degree seaweeds in the diet. However, it is the acetylated sugars (N-acetyl-glucosamine, N-acetyl-galactosamine and N-acetyl-neuraminic acid) that are so crucial for health and yet so hard to come by in meaningful amounts from any other sources than within animal connective tissues in our diet. This is why they are so commonly used as supplements in the form of glucosamine and galactosamine (found within chondroitin) for those with conditions requiring connective tissue support such as arthritic relief or in gut healing. It is therefore great to appreciate how a simple bone broth made from the cartilaginous bones of any healthy (preferably grass-fed) animal would contain all of these last three essential sugars in one highly palatable, powerful and affordable dietary supplement.

At this point it seems worth noting how many of our most essential nutrients for human health require whole and healthy animal sources, grown in chemical-free and mineral-rich soils. All things worth protecting for the wellbeing of ourselves, our loved ones and future generations seeking to live a happy and harmonious life into the ever-evolving future.

—Warren Maginn, functional clinical nutritionist

CHAPTER 11

Food as medicine

Back when I was studying for my degree in nutrition, I knew it felt like I was on the right path, but it wasn't until I completed two units entitled 'Food as Medicine' that I fell in love with what I was learning. Before then I only ever saw food as a number, a calorie, and I was hell bent on keeping that number as low as possible. I never cared about what was actually *in* the calories I was eating. I didn't care if it had nutrients, vitamins, minerals, essential fats—I was just interested in the number attached to the food and that was it. When I finished my 'Food as Medicine' units, my entire view on food and what it can do for health had completely changed.

Food is so much more than just food. The right food can heal you! Food can help you sleep better, improve your mood, stop you from getting colds, reduce your stress, improve your memory, reduce the effects of ageing, improve your joints, it can make your skin clear, your hair shiny and give you more energy. Phew! And that is just the start of it. It is magical, wonderful, powerful stuff, BUT you have to eat the right food. Do I have you excited? You should be!

Make your kitchen your very own pharmacy

Hippocrates, the father of medicine, said, 'Let food be thy medicine and medicine be thy food'—and this is what we have forgotten how to do.

We are losing touch with what real food looks like and where our food comes from. Jamie Oliver demonstrated this in his TV series *Jamie's Food Revolution,* where many school-aged children could not even recognise or name simple real foods such as beetroot or broccoli. It is a real tragedy that kids are growing up these days believing that all food comes from the supermarket and in packets. We have become so disconnected from the land and where our food is sourced. Do we really want our kids growing up thinking that a piece of steak is made in the supermarket?

Think about what you ate today. Do you know where your food came from? And I don't just mean the shop where you bought it! Think about it for a moment. How much do you actually know about what you eat or feed your family? The food that you put in your mouth every day has such a profound and important impact on YOUR health—what is in it, how it was processed, where it came from, and how was it grown. The origin of your food is very important.

So, what is the easiest way to set up your own kitchen pharmacy? Firstly, clean out all the junk foods from your cupboards. I don't believe in keeping them there for a special occasion. I am all for 'keeping it real' and realise that you are not likely to eat 100 per cent Paleo all of the time, but when switching to Paleo and undertaking the 28-day Reset protocol, there is no need to have temptation hanging around in the pantry. Get it all out and throw it away! You will feel much better for it.

Have a look at the seasonal produce list I have included at the end of this chapter—that is your perfect guide to creating your very own kitchen pharmacy. Mother Nature has done all the hard work for you! You see, when you eat seasonally, you change the foods you are getting all year round and therefore gain a broad variety of nutrients—your very own multivitamin!

Herbs! I love herbs! Stock your pantry with a huge variety of herbs and, if you can, some fresh home-grown ones. They not only add flavour to any meal, but also a massive amount of nutrients to your diet. Herbs are the little powerhouses of the plant kingdom, and are fantastic in aiding everything from supporting the immune system to reducing inflammation. I'll tell you more about some of my favourite herbs shortly.

Setting up your new pantry and kitchen may involve a small outlay of money, but it will be worth it. Keep in mind that you don't have to do it all at once; just add a new dried herb to your pantry every couple of weeks and before you know it, you will have a huge selection to draw from. The diversity of flavours you will experience will motivate you to keep going Paleo and the benefits to your health will save you from trips to the doctor.

The incalculable value of real food

'Now with more added omega-3' or 'contains three times more anti-oxidants' or 'now with added fibre'. How many times do you see these advertisements for packaged foods? We are starting to fortify everything that comes in packaging. Why? To make it healthy?

The other new kid on the market is a pill that promises to give you all the vitamins and minerals you need to meet the required daily intakes you would get from eating your fruit and vegetables—with the catchcry that trying to eat this amount of vegetables and fruit takes so much time and planning! Yes, hard work, isn't it? So, let's all just pop a pill instead, right? WRONG!

You can't out-do nature. The synergistic effect of real food is priceless. Scientists are now finding out that people taking a whole bunch of anti-oxidant supplements may actually be worse off than people not taking them. Why? Because taking a single extracted, heavily processed vitamin or mineral is not the same as getting that vitamin or mineral along with all the other cofactors (other vitamins or minerals that are needed for it to do its job properly) that it needs in order to perform the required function in the body. You see, all nutrients work together with a whole bunch of other nutrients in order to make things happen in the body.

There is a time and place for nutritional supplementation support, and as a practitioner I do use these supplementation therapies with my clients, but always combined with utilising food as medicine, as this is the real key when it comes to looking after your health.

Real food contains something I like to call 'a little bit of magic'. I am certain that what is in real food and what our body does with it is even more complex than what research has discovered to date. Scientists have tried to figure out why food is so good and replicate it, but our manmade versions just don't have the same effect as the 'magic' that is contained in real food.

We are more than the sum of our parts and so is our food. It is for this reason that we need to make sure that the way our plants and animals are grown, treated and looked after is in keeping with what will produce the most healthy, happy, high-quality food. That way all of the goodness gets passed on to us!

Free-range, wild, grass-fed meat

We thrive and have better health when we eat a diet that is conducive to our health and this is no different for any other animal. Animals, even domesticated ones, are not designed to eat processed food. They are not meant to eat soy meal, corn meal, protein meal or synthetic vitamins, and it is reflected in their health and the breakdown of nutrients available to us from consuming that animal.

Big industry always wants to make the quickest turnover for the least amount of outlay, which means feeding animals a grain-based diet. It fattens them up fast (giving them more pro-inflammatory omega-6) and is a cheap food source.

I'm a big believer in ethical farming. I like to know that the animal I am eating has had a healthy, sunshine-filled life and in doing so it will be passing on its healthy energy and nutrients to me.

Grass-fed means that the cows are eating what cows are meant to eat—grass. This gives their meat a much better omega-3 to omega-6 ratio and more nutrients, such as vitamin K2 and beta-carotene. The meat will be leaner (as the animal has not been unhealthily fattened up by grains) and the fat will be a yellowish colour from betacarotene (from eating the grass). The animal is healthier and does not need a lot of the synthetic nutrients and antibiotics that grain-fed animals may need.

Wild versus farmed fish is another consideration. Farmed fish are fed pellets, which means that they have a much lower omega-3 content and a much higher omega-6 content. Not good. Where possible, try to get your hands on some wild-caught fish. However, mercury levels in some wild fish also need to be considered, especially for pregnant women. Although swordfish has good levels of omega-3, it rates high for potential mercury contamination and should be limited. Great oily fish with low ratings for mercury contamination include anchovies, mackerel and sardines.

Vegetables and fruits

A raspberry is a just a raspberry, right? Well, yes, but I want you to always consider the *origin* of your foods, especially when it comes to fruit and vegetables. Where did your raspberries come from? Were they flown 10,000 kilometres to get to you? Can you eat raspberries at all times of the year? You might think you can judge by what is available in the supermarket, but in reality, it is a seasonal fruit.

Seasonal eating
Seasonal eating is something that I believe is rarely practised these days and I must admit that even I find I forget what is available when because when I go into the shops everything is available! Nearly every fruit and vegetable is available at all times of the year

in supermarkets and I think this is detrimental for a few reasons:

- Because we are disconnected from our land and where food comes from we don't actually know what is available in the seasons. We need to re-establish this connection with nature to understand seasonality.

- We do not eat enough of a variety of foods (and the nutrients from them), as we tend to stick to our 'likes' and not try anything new. When was the last time you tried a new fruit or vegetable?

- Our carbon footprint is so huge from transporting foods all over the world to meet this demand of having foods available all of the time and not just seasonally.

Eating seasonally is an easy way to get a great variety of nutrients because you mix it up with the seasons! Become a locavore (a person who actively seeks out local produce), so that you encourage food not to be moved thousands of kilometres to reach the market. It is a great way of eating and a good way to get the kids involved. You can make a game of it. Visit all the local markets and butchers and see what little gems you find—you will be surprised! And I promise you will love the price as well.

Eating organic
When it comes to eating fruits and vegetables, you will see a lot of debate going on as to whether you

should buy organic or not. One of the big issues surrounding organic is the price—and I completely understand this. We don't all have a lot of free cash and we want to know that what we are spending our money on is worth it.

My general rule of thumb goes like this: where possible, I first like to make sure that the meat I am buying is grass-fed, free-range and wild, and I am prepared to spend the money on that as I believe that is totally worth the price. When it comes to fruit and vegetables, I like to stick with trying to buy organic when it comes to the 'Dirty Dozen' and all the rest I am happy to just get from my local farmers' market.

The Environmental Working Group (EWG) have a list they put together every year of what they like to call the 'Dirty Dozen'—a list of fruit and vegetables that may carry pesticide residues. These are the guys that you want to try to buy organic. The EWG also have a 'clean' list, which lets you know the fruit and vegetables with the lowest risk of pesticide residue.

DIRTY DOZEN (BUY ORGANIC)

Apples

Spinach

Celery

Lettuce

Capsicum (peppers)

Cucumbers

Peaches

Blueberries

Strawberries

Potatoes

Nectarines

Grapes

(Source: www.ewg.org)

An easy way I like to look at this is that if you eat the outside skin, be a little cautious as to where you got the fruit or vegetable from and try for organic. If you generally cut off or peel the outer skin, you can be a little more relaxed as to the risk of pesticide residue, as you are taking off the outer layer.

You can also give your fruit and vegetables a rinse with a vinegar and water mix. I use one part apple cider vinegar to three parts water, either in a spray bottle or in the sink. Wash or spray the fruit and vegetables and then rinse off with water. I believe this helps as an antibacterial agent and removes some of the pesticide residue. It is easier to spray or briefly soak (for around 2 minutes) the harder skinned fruit and vegetables than the softer skinned types.

Food as medicine in practice

I just love, love, love food as medicine! Let's have a look at some of my favourite ways to use 'food as medicine'.

Mood foods

Raw cacao and dark chocolate (at least 85 per cent cacao)
- Cacao and dark chocolate are packed with anti-oxidants, which are essential when under periods of stress, as the stress response in the body produces higher levels of free radicals.

- Cacao and dark chocolate contain good levels of magnesium, which is highly beneficial during times of stress, as it gets used up at twice the rate during these periods.

- Magnesium is also helpful for muscle relaxation and is good for tight shoulders, necks, tension headaches and migraines.

Bananas, beef and pumpkin seeds
- All these foods are good for providing the body with the amino acid tryptophan, which is needed to make serotonin—your feel-good neurotransmitter (chemical signaller).

- Sweet cravings can increase the demand for tryptophan, so eating these foods will help.

Balancing hormones

Cauliflower, broccoli, brussels sprouts and cabbage

- All these foods are cruciferous vegetables and contain quantities of sulphur-containing phytochemicals such as sulforaphane and indole-3-carbinol (I3C).

- Oestrogens (there are actually three different principal forms of oestrogen) are primarily metabolised by the liver through phase I and phase II pathways and then they are excreted. Sulforaphane and I3C work on your phase II liver detox pathway, which is responsible for the safe clearing of oestrogen metabolites from your body.

- Excess oestrogen or oestrogen dominance is very common in women today and can be linked to PMS, polycystic ovary syndrome, heavy periods, cancers, ovarian cysts, weight gain, etc. So consuming these foods will assist with excess oestrogen clearance.

- Consumption of these foods, however, coupled with iodine deficiency, can exacerbate low thyroid conditions as they exert anti-thyroid activity and should be monitored.

Seaweed, asparagus and seafood

- Seaweed, asparagus and seafood are all good sources of iodine, which is needed for thyroid health. In 2009, the World Health Organization stated that iodine deficiency disorders affected 800 million people worldwide.

Brazil nuts, liver and mackerel

- All these foods deliver a good punch with regards to selenium. Selenium is also required for good thyroid function, and selenium deficiency is all too common today. Selenium deficiency is also linked to infertility in both men and women. So, if you want to make happy and healthy babies, get good levels of these foods into you!

Inflammation

Turmeric

- I just LOVE turmeric; it is one of my favourite foods! The active ingredient in turmeric is curcumin, which has been shown to be everything from anti-inflammatory to anti-ageing to anti-cancer. Turmeric is beneficial in so many ways, so start adding this amazing food to your diet today.

- Turmeric is most notably researched for its anti-inflammatory properties, with studies showing that it is a powerhouse anti-inflammatory by blocking the formation of cyclooxygenases (COX-2) and other pro-inflammatory messengers such as interleukin-1, interleukin-6, interleukin-8 and tumour necrosis factor alpha.

148

Ginger
- Ginger is another little power player in reducing inflammation. It helps reduce many of the pro-inflammatory messengers, as turmeric does, such as interleukin-1 and tumour necrosis factor alpha.

Onion, broccoli, apple and kale
- All these foods contain a flavonoid called quercetin, which has also been shown in studies to be a strong inhibitor of COX-2 and a powerful anti-inflammatory.

Immunity

Onion and garlic
- Both onion and garlic contain selenium, which is important for enhancing white blood cell production and protects the body from free radical damage. It is needed for maintaining resistance to disease and infection.

- Onions decrease phlegm and inflammation. They kill bacteria and can prevent infections.

- Garlic is Mother Nature's antibiotic! Garlic needs to be chopped to release its active ingredients, which then need to be consumed within a couple of hours. This is why it is so important to use freshly chopped garlic and not pre-chopped, jarred garlic.

- Garlic stimulates the immune system and prevents and relieves chronic bronchitis. It also acts as a decongestant, so it is great for clearing chesty colds.

Ginger
- Ginger contains zinc, which is essential for good immune system functioning.

- Ginger also minimises the symptoms of a cold or other respiratory conditions by dilating constricted bronchial tubes, because it is warming.

- It is wonderful to use fresh as a tea with honey and lemon to relieve sinus congestion.

Herbs
- Herbs contain a large amount of phytochemicals such as different carotenoids, which make them powerful immune boosters, helping to protect against colds and flu.

- They are also packed with anti-oxidants, vitamins and minerals, so are super good for you as well as adding super flavour to your dishes!

Although I have listed some of the active ingredients of individual foods here, a lot of the researchers still have not found the exact mechanisms for how these foods do what they do. I believe that this is again the synergistic effect of all of the nutrients in the food working together. Remember, you can't out-do Mother Nature.

Seasonal produce list

SPRING

Artichoke

Asparagus

Avocado

Banana

Blood orange

Broad beans (fava beans)

Broccoli

Cabbage

Carrot

Cauliflower

Cherry

Chives

Cucumber

Cumquat

Dragon fruit

Grape fruit

Honeydew melon

Kale

Leek

Lemon

Lettuce

Loquat

Lychee

Mandarin

Mango

Orange

Papaya (pawpaw)

Peas

Pineapple

Potato

Rhubarb

Rockmelon (cantaloupe)

Seville orange

Silverbeet (chard)

Snow peas (mangetout)

Spinach

Strawberry

Sugar snap peas

Sweetcorn

Tangelo

Tomato

Valencia orange

Watercress

Watermelon

Zucchini (courgette)

SUMMER

Apricot

Cucumber

Lychee

Rockmelon (cantaloupe)

Asparagus

Currant

Mango

Avocado

Dragon fruit

Mangosteen

Squash

Bamboo shoots

Eggplant (aubergine)

Mulberry

Star fruit

Banana

Gooseberry

Nectarine

Strawberry

Blackberry

Green beans

Okra

Sugar snap peas

Blueberry

Guava

Passionfruit

Sweetcorn

Borlotti beans

Honeydew melon

Peas

Tamarillo

Boysenberry

Kale

Pineapple

Tomato

Capsicum (peppers)

Kiwi fruit

Radish

Valencia orange

Celery

Leek

Rambutan

Watermelon

Cherry

Lettuce

Raspberry

Zucchini (courgette)

Chives

Loganberry

Rhubarb

Zucchini flower

AUTUMN

Apple

Custard apple

Mushrooms

Quince

Asian greens

Daikon

Nashi pear

Rhubarb

Avocado

Eggplant (aubergine)

Okra

Rockmelon (cantaloupe)

Banana

Endive (chicory)

Onion

Silverbeet (chard)

Beetroot (beets)

Fennel

Orange

Snow peas (mangetout)

Borlotti beans

Fig

Papaya

Spinach

Broccoli

Grapes

Parsnip

Spring onions (scallions)

Cabbage

Honeydew melon

Peach

Squash

Capsicum (peppers)

Kiwi fruit

Pear

Sugar snap peas

Carrot

Leek

Peas

Swede (rutabaga)

Cauliflower

Lemon

Persimmon

Sweet potato (kumara)

Celery

Lettuce

Plum

Sweetcorn

Chives

Lime

Pomegranate

Tomato

Cucumber

Mandarin

Potato

Turnip

Cumquat

Mango

Pumpkin

WINTER

Apple

Custard apple

Navel orange

Rhubarb

Asian greens

Endive (chicory)

Nuts

Silverbeet (chard)

Avocado

Fennel

Okra

Snow peas (mangetout)

Beetroot (beets)

Grapefruit

Olives

Blood orange

Horseradish

Onion

Spinach

Broccoli

Jerusalem artichoke

Parsnip

Spring onions (scallions)

Brussels sprouts

Kale Pear

Cabbage

Kiwi fruit

Peas

Sugar snap peas

Carrot

Leek

Persimmon

Swede (rutabaga)

Cauliflower

Lemon

Pineapple

Sweet potato (kumara)

Celeriac

Lime

Potato

Tangelo

Celery

Mandarin

Pumpkin

Turnip

Cumquat

Nashi pear

Quince

CHAPTER 12

You're not doing Paleo right unless you're eating more vegetables than a vegetarian!

How many times have you heard quoted in the media that the Paleo diet or Caveman diet is all about eating a high-meat diet? I hear it all the time and it drives me crazy! It is NOT an all-meat diet! And many of the negative factors people associate with the diet are linked to this misconception.

Let's get one thing straight—unless you eat more vegetables than a vegetarian, you are not doing Paleo right. And I REALLY mean this! Vegetables make up a very large portion of eating well and it is extensively documented that a diet high in plant matter (vegetables and fruit) will lead to lower disease rates. SO, EAT THEM UP!

Vegetables are literally powerhouses, jam packed with vitamins and minerals in an easy to digest form. Anti-oxidant, anti-cancer, antibacterial, anti-inflammatory, antiviral—you name it, vegetables help you out with it. Making the conscious effort to add them to your diet will do wonders for your health, your skin and your quality of life.

The cool thing is, and I have had this confirmed by many clients (even my husband, who is notorious for telling me the truth), when you cut out the excess, processed sugary junk from your diet—*vegetables taste AMAZING!* They really do. You will be happy eating a salad with no dressing on it (for real!) because the tomato tastes sweet, the cucumber is super juicy and things just simply taste so much better. You will learn to love eating your vegetables again—that is a promise.

Vegetables are powerhouses, jam-packed with vitamins and minerals. Anti-oxidant, anti-cancer, antibacterial, anti-inflammatory, anti-viral—you name it, vegetables help you out!

So, I want at least half (minimum requirement) of your plate filled with plant material, the other part with a portion of animal protein and add to that a little good fat and you're done, easy peasy!

Now that brings me to another myth that gets bandied around about Paleo. You hear a lot that you will not get enough fibre on this sort of template because you are missing the fibre from grains. To that I say, WRONG! If you follow the principle of eating more vegetables than a vegetarian, you will never have issues doing 'number twos'!

Most countries have values recommending how much nutrition a child or an adult should consume each day. The Nutrient Reference Values for Australia and New Zealand, set by the Australian Government, currently sit at 30g fibre per day for men and 25g fibre per day for women, to maintain a healthy gut.

As you can see from the following table, you will reach and even exceed this amount consuming a wide variety of seasonal vegetables and fruit in your daily diet. Listed are some examples of fruit and vegetables you may consume following this way of eating and you would possibly even consume more than this in one day.

AVERAGE CONSUMPTION PER DAY OF FRUIT AND VEGETABLES ON A PALEO TEMPLATE

FRUIT AND VEGETABLES	FIBER
1 cup cooked broccoli	5.2g
1/2 cup diced avocado	6g
1 cup cooked asparagus	3.6g
1 cup cooked cauliflower	2.8g
1 cucumber	1.5g
2 cups raw spinach	2g
1 cup raspberries	8g
1 cup cooked kale	3g
Total	32.1g

(Source: www.nutritiondata.self.com)

So, get excited about your vegetables (and fruit) and start getting adventurous—try different varieties you have not tasted before. Head down to your local farmers' markets and see what heirloom varieties they might have (heirloom fruit and vegetables are varieties that were grown in years gone by, before mass-producing agriculture). We used to have hundreds more varieties compared to the limited range you see in the supermarket today. Many of the heirloom fruit and vegetables were also not as sweet as the varieties we have today, and they don't look as 'pretty' as some store-bought versions, but they do offer different nutrient ratios and different tastes (some swear they taste better), so give them a go!

Another option is to try fruit and vegetables from different cultures. These days most developed countries are lucky to have access to a range of ingredients from other cultures. Here in Australia we are fortunate, because we have a multicultural society with an abundance of different foods. For example, I have local Asian grocers close to me where I can go and buy different exotic Asian fruit and vegetables.

You will find in traditional cultures, there is a special place for bitter, sour and pungent flavours, whereas in our Western culture, we are geared towards sweet, sweet and sweet! As I mentioned before, most of our fruit varieties have even been developed to be sweeter. We should learn to embrace bitter, sour and pungent flavours. Traditional cultures use these flavours for detoxifying and cleansing the internal organs and for stimulating digestion and metabolism.

Indigenous people can also have much to offer in the way of unique ingredients. For example, in Australia, indigenous foods are becoming a very popular choice for people to try. It's funny that many of the names include 'peaches', 'plums' and 'apples', because they were given the 'English equivalent' name based on their appearance, which imply they are sweet. But the reality is that they are anything but sweet! Nearly all of the indigenous Australian fruits are bitter and sour, which are common flavours for indigenous foods. Australian indigenous foods are packed with nutrients and have some of the highest levels of vitamins around. The wild plum found in eastern Arnhem Land has a vitamin C content of more than 50 times that of common citrus fruits—AMAZING!

The point is, get out there and be adventurous with your fruit and vegetables. There are so many more incredible flavours for you to discover!

CHAPTER 13

Good health starts in the gut

In Chapter 6 I described how our gut is like a delicate rainforest and if we want optimal health we really need to tend to this rainforest and keep it happy, healthy and in balance. But how do we keep our rainforest happy? Well, it's just like looking after a garden. You have to weed it, seed it and then feed it!

Leaky gut (increased intestinal permeability), an imbalance of gut bacteria and poor bowel health, can cause many sneaky signs and symptoms that you may not even associate with gut health, such as headaches, poor sleep, reduced concentration and fatigue.

A weed, seed and feed protocol is simply a way of reducing the assault on your gut from problematic foods and environmental toxins, in order to reduce inflammation and to heal the gut by providing it with the right nutrients and good bacteria to do so. It can be done in a very gentle manner, as I outline later in this chapter, and is a good way of 'spring cleaning' the gut every six months or so.

Have a look at the following quiz and see if any of the symptoms fit for you. They are some of the most common complaints I see in my clinic and they are all related to gut health.

GUT AND BOWEL HEALTH QUIZ CIRCLE ANY OF THE SYMPTOMS BELOW THAT YOU MAY EXPERIENCE ON A FREQUENT BASIS (2–3 TIMES PER WEEK)

Constipation or diar-rhoea	Reflux	Poor concentration
Frequent colds and flu	Irregular bowel move-ments	Excess mucus produc-tion
Allergies	'Floating' poo (it does not sink to the bottom of the toilet bowl)	Itching skin or rashes
Headaches	Hard 'pellet' poo	Acne
Joint pain	Burping or belching af-ter meals	Poor sleep
Bloating or gas	Food sensitivities	Changes in mood
Runny nose or post nasal drip	Cravings (especially sugar)	Fatigue

If you circled two or more symptoms, it is worth considering doing a Weed, Seed and Feed protocol.

Weed

It is time to weed your garden! This involves limiting or eliminating the assault on the gut barrier via external sources (e.g. problematic foods) and being on the lookout for any bacteria or pathogens that may have set up camp in your gut that should not be there. To do this:

- Remove processed sugars, refined foods, alcohol, grains, dairy and legumes from your diet and follow the 28-day Reset protocol (see Chapter 19).

- Reduce exposure to pesticides, insecticides and chemicals. Buy organic from the 'Dirty Dozen' (review from Chapter 11) and wash vegetables in the apple cider vinegar and water mix.

- The use of non-steroidal anti-inflammatories (NSAIDs), antibiotics, stress and high-intensity physical exercise can all contribute to the problem—so try to work on limiting these. You can reintroduce the high intensity exercise once you have repaired your gut.

Natural combinations of herbs such as black walnut, wormwood, rosemary, pau d'arco, barberry and garlic can all be used to help 'weed' due to their antimicrobial, antibacterial and anthelmintic (antiparasitic) properties. It is worth noting that these have very broad and indiscriminate ranges of action and you should seek the guidance of a trained nutritionist or naturopath who can help you identify which would be most appropriate for your situation (especially if you are pregnant or ill). This will help you avoid possibly creating further imbalances to your digestive system through guesswork.

Seed

What you 'plant' (good bacteria) in your garden is very important, but so is the 'soil' (gut lining), because unless that is healthy, your plants won't grow!

A healthy gut lining is essential for good gut health. During this time you want to utilise nutrients that will reduce inflammation and help to heal the gut lining. The following nutrients will set the path to good gut health:

- **L-glutamine:** This is an essential nutrient for enterocytes (cells in your gut) as it provides the fuel for these cells. Supplementation of L-glutamine can strengthen gut barrier function, reduce inflammation and enhance immunity.

- **EPA/DHA:** These omega-3s are essential for reducing inflammation (as seen in Chapter 10). Supplementation with a good fish oil is very beneficial during this time, as well as eating good quality oily fish. Choose a fish oil that is in triglyceride form, is processed in an oxygen-free environment, and derives from fish that were ethically caught.

- **Vitamin A:** Cod liver oil is great because it also contains natural levels of vitamin A, which has a role in cell integrity and maintaining a good gut barrier.

- **Zinc:** Important for the development of enterocytes, zinc is beneficial for reducing inflammation. It is a very common deficiency seen in today's society.

- **Curcumin and quercetin:** Both these nutrients are potent anti-inflammatories and help to dampen the inflammation cascade. Curcumin is also antimicrobial and helps to reduce intestinal permeability.

- **Glycine:** This is needed to heal from infection and inflammation. It aids detoxification and digestion. You can get good levels of glycine from bone broth, which is wonderfully healing on the gut.

- **Gentian, artichoke and barberry:** These are all 'bitter' herbs and aid digestion through promoting the secretion of digestive juices, helping the breakdown of nutrients and therefore reducing the possibility of larger particles gaining entry through the intestinal wall.

Prebiotics and probiotics

Prebiotics

Prebiotics are non-digestible carbohydrates that are fermented by gut bacteria into short-chain fatty acids. They can promote the growth of beneficial commensal bacteria, such as strains of *Lactobacillus* and *Bifidobacterium.* However, the ingestion of prebiotic foods and short-chain carbohydrates (fermentable oligosaccharides, disaccharides, monosaccharides and polyols—FODMAPs) can become an issue with people who have functional gut disorders (such as carbohydrate malabsorption), or conditions such as irritable bowel syndrome (IBS). The carbohydrates end up being fermented in the small intestine and can cause a bacterial overgrowth in this area known as 'small intestine bacterial overgrowth' (SIBO). Common symptoms of SIBO include cramping, gas, diarrhoea, constipation and abdominal pain.

> Poor digestion and low hydrochloric acid in the stomach can contribute to carbohydrate malabsorption and SIBO.

Poor digestion and low hydrochloric acid in the stomach to carbohydrate can contribute to carbohydrate malabsorption and SIBO, so adopting a low FODMAPs diet can be beneficial. Supplements containing prebiotics such as frutco-oligosaccharides (FOS), galato-oligosaccharides (GOS) and even apple pectin and slippery elm should be used with caution. They may increase symptoms associated with carbohydrate malabsorption such as bloating, pain and altered bowel movements and exacerbate SIBO. Common FODMAP foods to avoid include:

- **Fructans:** Artichokes (globe and Jerusalem), asparagus, beetroot, garlic, leek, onions, raddichio lettuce, spring onion, wheat, rye, inulin, FOS.

- **Lactose:** Most dairy such as milk, ice cream, custard, condensed milk, milk powder, yoghurt, margarine, soft cheeses.

- **Galacto-oligosaccharides (GOS):** Legume beans, lentils, chickpeas.

- **Polyols:** Apples, apricots, avocado, cherries, lychees, nectarines, pears, plums, prunes, mushrooms, sorbitol, xylitol, maltitol.

- **Foods that contain high fructose:** Agave, apples, honey, mango, pear, raisins, watermelon.

Because it is very common for people to have digestive issues, I do not generally recommend taking an actual prebiotic supplement, unless under the care of a professional who has recommended it. You do not generally eat whopping great amounts of FODMAP foods on Paleo, but just keep it in the back of your mind if you are still having gut issues and perhaps look at limiting them while you do a gut repair protocol and seek out the assistance of a nutritionist.

Probiotics

I'm sure by now most of you have heard about probiotics. They are bacteria that create lactic acid and are live microorganisms that are ingested to give you good levels of good bugs (friendlies) and help provide protection from the bad guys, keeping you in good health. They do this by improving your immune response, normalising intestinal permeability, and inhibiting pathogenic bacteria.

It is fairly safe to say that everyone could do with a dose-up of good bugs! We all suffer from stress (sometimes more than others), most of us have been on a course of antibiotics and we don't always have the perfect diet.

I believe that it is beneficial to get the assisted boost from a probiotic supplement during the time you are doing a 'seed' and then keep your gut happy with lots of good probiotic foods after that point. Then if you ever have an illness, are under lots of stress or have to have another course of antibiotics, top up with a supplementation course again. Although there are many different strains of bacteria, the ones generally used in probiotic supplementations belong to the *Lactobacillus* and *Bifidobacterium* genera.

> Supplement for a specific purpose and then switch to 'food as medicine' probiotic foods.

Probiotics have been shown to be strain-specific and therefore different strains are more beneficial than others for various conditions. See some of the examples opposite.

IMPROVE IMMUNITY	ANTIBIOTIC USE	IMPROVING GUT BARRIER FUNCTION AND ANTI-INFLAMMATORY
Lactobacillus rhamnosus GG	Bifidobacterium animalis subsp. lactis Bb12	Lactobacillus rhamnosus GG
Bifidobacterium animalis subsp. lactis Bi-07	Lactobacillus rhamnosus GG	Lactobacillus plantarum MB452

IMPROVE IMMUNITY	ANTIBIOTIC USE	IMPROVING GUT BARRIER FUNCTION AND ANTI-INFLAMMATORY
Bifidobacterium lactis HN019	Lactobacillus reuteri MM53	Lactobacillus plantarum DSM 2648

Find a good multi-strain probiotic and make sure the count of microorganisms is in the billions per capsule. I like multi-strains because single strains can tip the scales of a particular bacteria strain over another. Take the recommended dosage on the bottle, but have it on an empty stomach, away from food. I also do not think it is necessary to take them all the time. Supplement for a specific purpose and then switch to 'food as medicine' probiotic foods, which I have listed below.

Feed

Once you have weeded your garden and planted a good bed of bugs, you need to keep them watered and well. This is practising good preventative medicine and it comes in the form of having good probiotic foods every day, as well as continuing an anti-inflammatory diet. Probiotic foods are foods (and drinks) that have been fermented by using a process called lacto-fermentation.

In many traditional cultures, fermented foods are a staple and for good reason! Western cultures used to also consume more fermented foods than we do today. Who remembers their Gran pickling her vegetables?

This is what we need to get back to—eating fermented foods as a part of our everyday life. It keeps you healthy by providing good gut bacteria, while making the foods more digestible and providing beneficial enzymes.

- Sauerkraut and kimchi are dishes made by fermenting vegetables. Sauerkraut usually has a base of cabbage, while kimchi has napa cabbage and radish as its main ingredients and it is usually spicy hot. There are hundreds of different versions of both dishes.

- Kefir is a fermented milk drink and kombucha is made by fermenting tea (usually a black or green tea). Kombucha can undergo a second fermentation, where flavour can be added using various herbs or fruits such as berries. This produces a bubbly, almost soda-like drink.

- Yoghurt is fine if you can tolerate dairy, but make sure it is full fat, pot set and free from artificial flavours and sugar. Pot-set yoghurt is made by putting milk and a bacteria culture in individual containers, where it is then sealed and incubated. This produces the highest probiotic counts, which is exactly what you want. Alternatively, you could make your own. I make coconut cream yoghurt, which is a great dairy-free version.

Keep in mind that if you are new to fermented foods take it slow! The symptoms that are associated with gastrointestinal upset (bloating, gas, pain, diarrhoea) can also be caused by the addition of too many fermented foods in a short space of time. Start with a tablespoon every second day and slowly build up from there.

Good gut health starts young

In Chapter 6 I touched on the fact that a baby's development of good bacteria is paramount for their development. It is also essential for building their immune defences. Remember, a baby who has been delivered by caesarean section or who has been bottle-fed, has a greater risk of developing asthma and food allergies later in life. Studies have also shown that low numbers of *Lactobacillus* and *Bifidobacterium* are linked with fussing and crying in early infancy. To support the development of good bacteria in a baby's intestinal tract:

- It can be beneficial for a mother to be on a probiotic supplement while breastfeeding, as the good bugs get passed on to the baby.

- Babies can benefit from being on a specifically formulated probiotic supplement that also contains a prebiotic, to stimulate the growth of beneficial bacteria.

- Special consideration should be given to additionally supplement babies who have been delivered by caesarean section or who are being bottle-fed.

- A course of probiotics would benefit a baby or child who has been on a course of antibiotics. Make sure the probiotic is specifically formulated for children.

- Cod liver oil at a formulated dose for babies is also perfect for building up a little one's immune system and gut integrity.

Feeding your bugs should become part of your daily ritual for good health. It is not something that you should do just once and then forget about. Love your bugs!

CHAPTER 14

Calorie counting, dieting and intermittent fasting

As humans we always seem to want the black-and-white scientific answers to things, especially when it comes to nutrition and foods. But you know what? Sometimes, that is just not possible. I think this 'wanting all the answers' has led to us no longer trusting our natural instincts or the messages we get from our body. We seem to equate difficulty with somehow being superior and simplicity with being too simple to work—too simple to be true! We want to know the calories in a certain food, what portion to eat, when to eat it and how to cook it. Heaven forbid someone would just tell us to eat real food! We have forgotten what came naturally to us in the past.

Calorie counting

What is a calorie? A calorie is defined as the amount of energy needed to raise the temperature of 1 gram of water by 1 degree Celsius. Makes sense, right? So how do we measure calories in food? With a bomb calorimeter! Scientists put a portion of a food into the bomb calorimeter and burn the food (which is in an inside chamber), while measuring the temperature rise in the water (which is in an outer chamber). The final water temperature will give the 'calories' in a particular food.

My issue with this is that we do not burn food; we digest and assimilate nutrients. Further to that, our bodies are individual, we all have different digestion functionality, different loads on our immune system, different gut flora, etc. Do we all obtain the same amount of energy from a particular food? No, we don't. So why get all caught up measuring it?

> When you eat a diet that is full of nutrient-dense foods, with limited or no processed junk ... you don't need to weigh, count or track foods.

It also stops us looking at food as being a 'natural' thing. We start looking at food in terms or numbers and figures as opposed to what nourishment this food can give us. Food QUALITY means a lot more than food CALORIES!

When you eat a diet that is full of nutrient-dense foods, with limited or no processed junk, your body's own natural signalling will tell you when you are full and when you need to eat again. Eating seasonally will add variety to this and help deliver a wide range of nutrients. Trust this process. You don't need to weigh, count or track foods.

Let me reiterate. When you're eating real food your body will tell you when you've had enough, and when

180

you haven't. There is no other animal on this earth that feels the need to measure out its food. So, why should we?

Dieting

Dieting is such a dirty word these days! Even the word 'diet' has negativity attached to it. In the world of nutritionists, 'diet' is a word used to describe how an individual eats, not necessarily a proposed way of eating intended to aid weight loss. For the purpose of this chapter, however, when I refer to 'dieting' I will be referring to a way of eating intended to aid in weight loss.

Most of us have been on a diet, or know someone who has. There are hundreds of diets to choose from—shakes, meal replacements and meal deliveries—and its a multi-million dollar industry.

When did 'we' as a human race need to start dieting? Did it start with the advent of processed foods? Did it start when we began to 'mess' with what used to be 'real food'?

If you have tried a diet that involved calorie restriction, packaged food (usually low fat) or meal replacements, did it work? Did you fall off the bandwagon? Chances are you either stopped the diet and gained your weight back, or violated your diet and gained your weight back. Don't feel bad, there are research articles to back you up, so you are not alone and this happens to a lot of people. We are not designed to live off shakes or calorie-restricted diets and the moment we stop or go back to eating 'food' all of the weight comes back again—and usually with the addition of more than before!

Diets do not work! There is no quick fix or miracle diet. Eating using a Paleo template allows you to eat in a way that is sustainable for you, while rebalancing your weight and your hormones. It is not a fad diet; it is a simple way of eating that combines the most nutrient-dense foods available, while eliminating problematic foods for an individual. Sometimes simple is best and simple is that easy!

Intermittent fasting

Intermittent fasting (IF) is the practice of deliberate periods of fasting, alternated with periods of feeding. It has been used worldwide for a long time by various traditional, cultural and religious groups—most notably the Islamic fasting ceremony of Ramadan, where Muslims do not eat or drink during daylight hours. Although it has been used in traditional cultures for many years, IF is fast becoming the go-to method for improving your bio markers (insulin sensitivity, cholesterol levels, etc.), to help you lose those stubborn few kilos of weight, or even to extend your life.

Is intermittent fasting beneficial?

Short answer—yes and no! As is the case with everything to do with health and the body, it depends on the individual, and it is a topic so complex an entire book should be written about it!

IF can be considered anything from skipping a meal, to a condensed window of eating (consuming your daily food intake in a reduced number of hours), to extended (longer than 24 hours) fasts. Generally, IF follows a 'feast period' and then a 'fast period' so that usually the normal calorie count is still consumed, although sometimes that is not the case. There are many different programs outlining how and when this should be timed, and this will affect the outcome for an individual.

Not surprisingly, the body shows adaptive biochemical and physiological responses to the lack of food during the 'fast period' and it is about assessing whether those responses for an individual are going to assist or hinder their health. Potential health benefits can include:

- Improved insulin sensitivity.
- Reduced inflammatory markers.
- Reduced pain sensitivity.
- Weight loss.
- Improved cholesterol and triglyceride levels.

- Improved glucose tolerance (particularly in men).

- Improved hormonal responses, such as insulin sensitivity and glucose tolerance, while reducing cardio risk factors for obese individuals.

Potential negative health effects include:

- Weight gain.

- Hormonal imbalances (particularly reproductive hormones).

- Increased cortisol release.

- Increased chronic stress.

- Reduced quality of sleep.

- Possible adverse effects on glucose tolerance for non-obese individuals.

Keep in mind that IF does trigger a stress response in the body. So if you suffer from stress and anxiety in your life (which at times, can be all of us), then it would not be the best thing for you to do. You need to be fat adapted (using fat as your main energy source, not carbohydrates), have balanced hormones, and be sleeping well to do this. So in an everyday scenario, again it might not be the best thing to try.

However, there is a difference between skipping a meal because you are genuinely not hungry and a planned IF. I think it is quite healthy and sensible to listen to your body and only feed it when it is giving you the correct signals and not just mindlessly eating food because you always eat at 7a.m., 12p.m. and 8p.m. Start becoming more in tune to what your body is telling you.

You can see from the pros and cons listed above that anything is possible with IF! It can be good for your health and not so good for your health. It is about seeing what works for you as an individual, and I would suggest not attempting an IF program until you have discussed it with your naturopath, nutritionist, integrative GP or primary healthcare professional.

CHAPTER 15

Discovering a whole mind, body and soul connection

Lifestyle plays a very important role in health and gets overlooked a LOT! So many people concentrate on one aspect of health, say, looking after their diet, but they are stressed to the eyeballs, don't sleep and don't exercise! Healthy? No. Others might be exercising religiously, but they are forgetting all of the other aspects related to health. It is a whole mind, body and soul connection. It sounds hippie, but really it isn't! We have already seen in the previous chapters that what you eat can affect your biochemistry—which can affect your mood—which can affect your physical body. It's all connected and you really need to put the effort into balancing all three. Science is now catching up with this connection and more studies are coming out showing the importance of keeping a good balance in life.

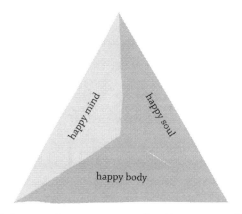

good health is the sum of all parts in balance

Our lifestyles have changed drastically over the past 50 years and I don't think that they have changed for the better. We are sleep deprived, we have teenagers suffering from social media withdrawal and we are more stressed than ever. Technology has given us so much advancement in the world of health, but it is also stealing away our quality of life AND our health.

I want to go over some ways that can help you to bring back that balance to your mind, body and soul.

Sleep

We know sleep is important, yet so many of us still do not get enough. Please, above all else, make it a priority! I have already shown you that even just one night of sleep deprivation can reduce your leptin levels and elevate your ghrelin levels.

Poor sleep is also associated with hypertension, obesity, insulin resistance, poor immunity, depression, impaired glucose regulation, emotional instability, decreased cognitive function, stroke, heart disease and diabetes. Do I need to mention anymore? Sleep is SO important! Please make it the number one priority it deserves to be.

Repeat after me: *sleep is the most important thing to me; sleep is the most important thing to me!*

How do you get a good night's sleep?

This is where it will take some commitment on your behalf, as some of these changes will involve breaking bad old habits. It is worth making these changes as part of your 28-day Reset protocol (outlined in Chapter 19), but any small change is a step in the right direction, so see if you can implement one tonight!

Keep regular sleep and wake cycles, even on the weekends

Sometimes this is easier said than done, but keeping regular sleep-and-wake cycles will really help you, especially if you have issues getting off to sleep. Sleeping-in excessively on the weekends can disrupt a good sleep pattern. I aim to get to bed around 9.30p.m. to 10p.m. every night. Yep, you heard me, 9.30p.m.! This is an optimal time to be getting to bed. Try it out and see how much better you feel!

Create a regular bedtime ritual

This is also helpful for people who find it difficult to get to sleep. Listen to some soft music or take a warm bath or shower. Just try to make it your 'relaxing' preparation time before bed. Meditation or deep breathing can also help you to relax before bedtime. A ritual I love to practise is going to bed thinking about three good things that happened during the day. It helps you to see the positive side of life (even after a bad day) and lets you fall asleep with your mind in a happy place.

Create a room conducive to good sleep

Your room needs to be dark and quiet, so remove any electrical gadgets that emit light and keep you active. Smart phones, tablets, laptops and TVs should all be banned from the bedroom! Your bed should only be used for sleep and lovin'—not surfing the web! Make sure you have a good mattress and pillow and keep the room on the slightly cooler side of things, as this helps you to sleep better.

Avoid caffeinated drinks after lunch

We know caffeine is a stimulant and its effects can be long lasting. That is why it's always safer to have your last caffeinated drink before lunch and then no more.

Avoid bright lights, intense activities and exercise before bedtime

Bright lights (including those from TVs, computer monitors and household lighting) affect our hormonal signalling that helps us sleep. Melatonin levels rise at night when it gets darker and our cortisol levels drop—all helping us to get to sleep. Increased light and stimulation, however, keeps cortisol elevated and prevents us from getting a good night's sleep. In particular, it is the blue rays in the lights that are the issue. Using blue light blocking glasses can assist with limiting light stimulation. I like to start turning off all of the gadgets we are using from about 8p.m. and begin to unwind. Exercise is best done in the early afternoon to avoid getting a cortisol spike too close to bedtime.

Exercise (play) and nature

I remember when I was a kid, Mum used to tell my sister and me to go outside and 'play'. She never told us to go outside and 'exercise'—but that is what we are telling today's generation of children. Yes, exercise is good for us and, yes, it has many health benefits, but is it fun? The thing is, if you really hate the type of exercise you are doing, are you going to continue to do it in the long run? Probably not. So find something that you like to do, something that you will stick with. That is the key! Not some form of exercise that is guaranteed to give you results but that you will only do for a month!

> I don't really care what you do! Just move, play and have fun.

Exercise can be a little bit like a double-edged sword. Why? Because it can actually cause some pretty severe hormonal disruptions—thyroid and cortisol are two examples. As I have briefly touched on before, exercise can induce a stress response in the body, which causes cortisol to be released and you go into 'flight or fight' mode. Now, as you found out in Chapter 5, most of us already have too much stress in our lives and it can potentially lead to some nasty health issues—leaky gut, for example. And exercise is supposed to relieve stress, right? Well, yes, it can do that, but this is where that pesky little word 'balance' comes up again. Don't overdo it! If you are super stressed, go for a walk instead of a 10-km run. Extremely strenuous exercise and overtraining doesn't help you or your health at all. A small study by Hackney et al. showed that high-intensity interval training (HIIT) suppressed the conversion of T4 to T3 (thyroid hormones) and that sufficient recovery time is needed for hormone levels to return to normal.

Find your fun factor!

I am sure you will be able to find research to back up every form of exercise out there and you will always hear about the latest fitness craze—high-intensity interval training (HIIT), cardio, running, weights, Crossfit, etc. They are all good forms of exercise and they all work, but I really want you to make a lifestyle change and move because you lIKE to move. I am not going to tell you what you should be doing, just get out there and move. And do it on a regular basis! Move because you have found something that you actually like to do. Try a whole lot of different things, see what suits you and what you like. Make it fun! Go rock climbing, go dancing, play soccer, go running, climb trees or do yoga—I don't really care what you do! Just move, play and have fun while you are doing it. It really is that simple. Any form of movement is good movement. I am not an exercise physiologist, but I do know that getting out there and moving is great for your body, mind and soul.

Make time to play! Schedule it into your diary and make an effort to do it as scheduled throughout the 28-day Reset protocol (see Chapter 19). Then notice the difference. You will be astounded by how much it positively affects all aspects of your life.

The power of nature

> *Given that our modern ways of living, as prescribed by Western industrialised culture, stand in stark contrast to our evolutionary history, it is proposed that we may currently be witnessing the beginnings of significant adverse outcomes for the human psyche.*—Eleonora Gullone, psychologist

Our environment has an influence on our psychological, physical and social wellbeing—something that we are only just starting to recognise.

People go to parks and gardens to sit among the trees, or go down and put their feet in the sand and listen to the ocean and find themselves feeling relaxed and at peace. Why? Because humans have an innate affinity towards nature—it's called biophilia. The trees and water keep us healthy!

Modern cities and our way of life are now dominated by manmade structures, technology and high-stress environments. This is a big change to the way we used to live as hunter– gatherers, when we used to live very closely with nature. The hypothesis of biophilia is that our affinity with nature is inherent in the way our nervous system develops. It is a part of us and being in and around nature makes us feel comforted and reassured.

Our current way of living is said to be an evolutionary mismatch and can be detrimental to our health. Researchers are now looking at how our discord with nature is adversely affecting our health and might be contributing to rates of obesity, depression, anxiety and stress. You know, it's even been shown that people recover better from surgery and ask for less pain medication when they have a lovely view of nature from their bedside window, compared to a view of a wall.

Spending time in nature can also improve behaviour, enhance cognitive function, reduce stress and have a restorative effect. If you add animals into the mix, say a dog, it also increases social interaction among humans.

Nature is where we all come from, what we are made of. We are nature.—Erwan Le Corré, founder of MovNat.

So, what do we do with this knowledge? We need to recognise the importance of nature and the positive role it plays in keeping us healthy. Make time to get out in nature, to feel the sand between your toes and to breathe in some salty air. It's very important for our health, especially if we live in a busy city. Even just putting more green plants in a room has been shown to reduce stress and increase feelings of wellbeing.

There are lots of small changes you can make to your life to improve your connection with nature. You could change your run route to include a park and not just main roads. You could add more shrubs to your backyard, have some potted plants in your house or make time on the weekends to get 'lost' in some natural bushland. What are you going to do to get more of Mother Nature in your life?

Nurturing relationships

Relationships are another aspect to 'whole health' that a lot of people forget about. Relationships can make us sick or they can make us healthy. When I talk about relationships, I am not just talking about romantic relationships, I am talking about every interaction we have—with both humans and animals.

Human beings are highly social creatures, but in our technology-driven world, we are losing the art of communication and nurturing relationships. We used to eat around a family table and talk over dinner, now we sit in front of the TV and zone out. We used to know our neighbours, but nowadays many people do not even know who lives next to them. We used to make time to catch up with our friends and discuss life, now we Facebook or Tweet them. It is all very superficial and we are living in a very isolated world, especially in big cities.

People with good social networks have fewer healthcare visits and spend less money on health care. People who have frequent face-to-face contact with friends have lower rates of depression. Being social and nurturing relationships KEEPS US Well!

Touch is another important aspect to nurturing relationships. It is not uncommon for humans to touch, even on first meeting. It might be a handshake, a hug or some other gesture of touch. It is reassuring, opens communication and sustains social bonds.

Touch or hugging, however, is often confused with things of a sexual nature, which is a misconception, but it has infiltrated our society. We do not hug as much anymore, which is sad because hugging and touch is innately human and is so beneficial for our health—it is healing. When babies are not touched they develop 'failure to thrive'. As adults, we still crave this human touch. Hormones such as oxytocin are released, which help to further enhance trusting, social bonds. A good hug can reduce your stress, get you out of a bad mood, make you feel acknowledged and be wonderfully reassuring.

In our busy, technologically advanced world, it is easy to forget the little things and not reach out and develop good social networks. It is, however, important to your health. So go and give your friends a good old-fashioned hug!

Reducing stress

Stress. There's a lot of it about and you know from Chapter 5 how damaging it can be to your health. So, how do you manage your stress? Well, there are many techniques you can implement in your life that will help you to better handle your stress. Simply incorporating everything I have just talked about earlier in this chapter will work wonders:

- Sleep well.

- Move daily.

- Get out in nature.

- Nurture your relationships.

- Other techniques you might want to try include:

  - **Meditation:** This relaxation technique has been shown to reduce physiological stress responses. A great way to start is with some guided CDs.

• **Qigong exercise:** This is the practice of aligning breath, movement and awareness. It is fantastic for reducing stress and improving feelings of wellbeing.

• **Diaphragmatic breathing:** This technique is full belly breathing. It can reduce stress and is great for enhancing relaxation. It is SO simple and so underutilised! It is a wonderful tool to incorporate into your night-time routine—simply take three long, deep breaths right before you are about to go to sleep to help you relax.

CHAPTER 16

Going Paleo

Remember how I said, 'My version of Paleo is not your version of Paleo and vice versa'? Well, it is important to understand that we are all unique and what my body will thrive on or be able to tolerate may be different to you.

I am big on empowering people to make choices for themselves. You should not blindly listen to or follow any health guru or expert. Do your own research and find out for yourself what works best for you regarding your health. Hold your own little n=1 experiment! Only you know your body and only you know what works best for you. One thing I believe all people need to do, however, is start with a blank canvas—and you can only do that after completing some sort of elimination protocol.

People think that following a Paleo template is some sort of new fad diet, but the practice of elimination diets has actually been around for a long time and that is essentially what Paleo is—an elimination diet that has options for the re-introduction of certain foods. Before I learnt about the Paleo template, one of the first things I nearly always did with my new clients was put them on an elimination protocol to assess if there were any hidden food triggers for the symptoms or conditions they presented with. When you get rid of problem foods you will be amazed how many little niggly things that you just always lived with, such as headaches, a runny nose, bloating and achy joints, will go away. They are not just a part of 'you' and you should not have to just live with them! They are your body's way of telling you that something is amiss.

An elimination diet involves stripping away all of the processed, highly allergenic and inflammatory foods in our diet for a designated period of time, so that we have a clean slate to work with. That way you can begin to recognise which foods your body has issues with and which foods it doesn't. That is, in essence, the beginnings of a Paleo template: a nutrient-dense way of eating that reduces or eliminates potential allergens and inflammatory foods. The rest is just about figuring out what works for you and your body.

Pressing the reset button

Pressing the reset button is an elimination protocol. It can be utilised by a newbie who is thinking about switching to a Paleo way of eating or someone who has been eating this way for a while but feels as though they are slipping a bit and falling back to some unhealthier food choices. It is also great for assisting gut repair as you eliminate inflammatory foods.

Why does a reset work?

It generally takes about 28 days for you to form new habits and develop new tastebuds, so it makes sense to commit to the reset for a period of 28 days, to allow you to start fresh. It also allows your body time to detoxify from the foods you were eating in the past, giving you that clean slate to work with, so you can see which foods you were previously eating that were affecting your health in a negative manner. It also allows time for inflammation to begin to settle down, the gut to begin to heal, and time for you to develop a new relationship with your food.

Why would you need to do a reset more than once?

Let's all acknowledge that we live in the real world. Life can sometimes get away from us, at different times we might be under huge amounts of stress and things just happen. You may be burning the midnight oil and not getting enough sleep or you had a serious relationship breakdown—any number of things! This may result in you eating a few too many takeaway dinners or indulging in a few too many glasses of wine. Perhaps you have discovered one of the hundreds of Paleo dessert blogs out there and you have been making a few too many of those. Yes, a dessert is a dessert, and you can even have too many Paleo ones!

These are all perfect reasons to do another reset protocol. Get your body back in check; get things back on track.

Essentially, the 28-day Reset protocol is a Paleo template minus all the 'grey' foods that individuals might not tolerate or else have an attachment to. Foods such as dairy (even raw dairy), pseudo-grains, beans and legumes all fall under this 'grey' foods category—as do desserts or snacks containing sweeteners (even natural ones), such as maple syrup or honey. Everyone can overindulge in these foods from time to time, and doing the 28-day Reset is about bringing your body back into balance. It is about enjoying real, nutrient-dense foods with no calorie restrictions and giving your body time to heal and get off the sugar-hit cycle.

What else should you do while undertaking the 28-day Reset?

This is also the perfect time to make some lifestyle changes! Just as at times our diet can slip, so can our lifestyle and we end up doing things that are not necessarily good for our health. I know I have stayed up late at night watching some rubbish on TV that I was barely interested in. This sort of thing does nothing for our health and, as we now know from Chapter 15, our sleep is very, very important for good health.

We all have busy lives and sometimes it is very easy to forget the simple things that can have such an impact on our overall health. Going to bed early, getting out into nature, relaxing, reducing stress, having fun and nurturing healthy relationships—this is what life should be about. People concentrate on these sorts of lifestyle changes when they have been diagnosed with cancer or something very serious, and it is amazing how many of these people are able to greatly help themselves to heal. Which begs the question: why are we not concentrating on these lifestyle changes now? Especially when it could help to PREVENT these sorts of health concerns in the first place! Do not underestimate the positive effect they will have on your life. Remember, sometimes the simplest things have the biggest impact.

CHAPTER 17

You only get out what you put in

This is where you have to endure a little tough love. You see, I am not going to sugar coat anything for you; switching over to Paleo or doing the 28-day Reset protocol is going to take some time and effort to complete. It is not always going to be hard, but making the initial changeover may be a little testing. So what's the key? Preparation and planning!

We plan for big events in our life, we plan at work and we plan for our holidays, yet not many of us seem to plan for our health. I know 'planning our health' sounds funny, but really, a little preparation in this area will have a profound, rippling effect throughout your life, both now and into the future. Who doesn't want to feel well, live long and be happy? We all do! But we won't find it by sitting back, popping a pill and eating junk. You only get out what you put in!

Weekly meal planning

When you first start Paleo, it is a good idea to devise weekly meal plans to help you stick to the template.

I sit down and plan what we are going to eat for the coming week, before we do the shopping on the weekend. This list goes up on the fridge and that way, everyone knows what is being made and whoever is in the kitchen first that night can see what is up on the list and start to prepare dinner. It does not need to be an exact recipe for each meal—I might even just write 'chicken and salad'. It just gives you an *idea* of what is to be made. What you decide on the night to actually put in the salad is up to you. If you want, and if it works for you, write down exactly what you want to make. Include the recipe book and page number, so you know which recipe to refer to on the night.

Weekly meal planning is also a good way to save money and stop you 'impulse buying' at the shops. Go in with your list, buy only what is on there and get out again! This also saves you from the 'what to have for dinner?' game. You know that game, when you have come home from a long day at work and you have nothing in mind for dinner and it all becomes too hard and you end up buying takeaway!

Commitment

To go Paleo and to improve your health, you need to *want* to change. There are habits that you are going to have to change in order to lead a healthier life and some of these habits might be hard to break, like staying up late and watching TV or surfing the internet. Lifestyle changes are just as important as food changes.

I hear people so often say that they do not have time to make a cooked breakfast in the morning. Well, guess what? You have two choices: you can set the alarm half an hour earlier in order to MAKE the time or you can do what my sister does. She's not a morning person, so she always cooks and prepares breakfast the night before, while she is making dinner. Then when she gets up for work the next day, her breakfast is ready to heat and eat. It just takes a bit of commitment.

Perhaps you are not used to cooking—it can be daunting at first. Stick with it because it does get easier and you will get quicker and come up with your own shortcuts for different things as time goes by. You just need to be committed.

Diet, emotions, reactions and responses diary (The DERR diary)

It may seem a bit odd to be keeping a food and mood diary, but it comes in really handy for figuring out things that may just be staring you in the face! This is why I call it the DERR diary, because you end up having a lightbulb moment and saying, 'Oh derr, now I see it!'

Keeping a DERR diary enables you to figure out which foods suit you and which ones don't. I mean this for both emotional attachments and gut reactions to foods. It will allow you to see what your trigger foods are and you will know how to handle them better. It is also a good way to get 'real' and honest with yourself, when you write down exactly what you eat. It is a great tool for a nutritionist or naturopath to pinpoint issues if you need to see them about something. This is where I can most commonly see that people are actually not eating enough.

After every meal or at the end of the day, just jot down:

- What you ate and if you had issues with cravings, hunger, etc.

- How your stomach handled the meal and whether there were any reactions, such as gas, pain, bloating, etc.

- Your stress levels out of 10 and reasons for the stress.

- Your mood out of 10 and how you are feeling.

You don't need to do this forever, but it is a great way to reconnect with yourself, your feelings and your foods. You will start to notice subtleties that you would not have noticed before and this is simply because you are actively bringing them to your own attention.

CHAPTER 18

Planning to succeed

I think the biggest point I can make about preparing for a change to Paleo or doing the 28-day Reset protocol is not to make the changeover in a time of severe stress. It takes work and careful planning and it should not be an 'added' stress in an already stressful situation. This is not to say that you are allowed to continually use stress as an excuse to NOT start! All I am saying is that you should wisely pick your time to make the switch. This means that contemplating a switch to Paleo while moving house is not a very good idea! Some helpful tips to start preparing to go Paleo include:

- Get organised over a weekend; it's worthwhile to devote some proper time to it. Just waking up on a Monday morning and hoping to start then and there is not good planning.

- Tell your family and friends what you are doing. That way you can enlist their support with the changes you are going to make. If you are doing the 28-day Reset protocol, tell them everything that is non-negotiable for this period of time. Let them know exactly what you can and cannot eat and ask them to respect your choices.

- Prepare your kitchen and pantry. Sort out which foods need to immediately go in the bin (e.g., processed junk or items not on the Paleo list) and what foods might need to be sectioned off for your n=1 experiments later.

- Photocopy the meal plan template from Chapter 19 or have some fun creating your own.

- Decide how you are going to write your DERR diary. Are you going to write notes in a journal or make your own daily template and photocopy it so you have enough copies to get you through the 28 days?

- Stock your kitchen and pantry with Paleo staples as outlined in Chapter 8. You can find pantry items such as coconut aminos (soy sauce replacement) and coconut butter at your local health food shop or online.

Kitchen gadgets for Paleo cooking

There are a few bits and pieces that make Paleo cooking that much easier, especially when you are making a lot of things from scratch. There are also a few 'Paleo' gadgets that you may not have used before, but you will learn to love them now! Here are some of my kitchen favourites:

- A good set of pots and pans, especially one really large stock pot to make big batches of bone broth and soups.

- Glass Pyrex containers. I use these ALL the time for food storage instead of plastic. It also means I can make extra meals and store them in the freezer. They can then go straight in the oven or microwave.

- Dehydrator—essential for making jerky, vegetable chips or fruit leather, although they are a bit of an investment. You can also make do with using your oven on a low heat and with the door slightly ajar.

- Mandolin slicer and julienne peeler. These little gadgets will make vegetable chips and zucchini noodles oh-so-much easier to make.

- Invest in a good blender, as you tend to get what you pay for with blenders. One that has a good speed and multiple blades will work wonders when creating nice smoothies and sauces.

- I also love a good hand blender. They are great for small jobs like making mayo or dukkah.

- A food processor. They are awesome for making quick meals. They chop a lot of things fast and can cut your prep time in half.

- Salad spinner—I never knew how fantastic they were until I got one! It allows you to wash your salads and then spin all the moisture out of them so that your lovely salad does not go soggy.

Fresh produce

Fresh is always best when it comes to produce, but this does not mean you have to grow your own. Don't get me wrong, it's awesome if you do grow your own produce, but I know that many people out there just do not have the time or space (or the will) to grow their own produce—me included! I do not have a green thumb!

> Get out in the community, get your hands dirty and share in locally produced foods.

You can, however, become a locavore and seek out local produce that is fresh, in season and cheap. This also means that the produce has not been moved thousands of kilometres to get to you and you are doing your bit to help the environment and reduce your carbon footprint! You can easily look up local farmers' markets and butchers on the internet to find out which ones are close to you.

Many more butchers now carry grass-fed beef; you just need to phone them and ask. Grass-fed beef is sometimes sold as one-quarter cow or half a cow. Sounds a bit odd talking about meat as a 'cow' but that is really what it is—well, when we are talking about beef! We have just become so disconnected from the origins of our meat. Buying meat like this is a great way to save money and become familiar with various cuts of meat you may not have bought in the past, as you get selections of all cuts and not just steaks. It is also a great way to slowly introduce yourself to 'nose-to-tail' eating.

Nose-to-tail eating was the way our grandmother used to eat and is the way a lot of traditional cultures still eat. We are so used to having premium cuts of meat these days that we forget about all the 'other bits' that now go to waste. The benefits of nose-to-tail eating are:

- You are not wasting perfectly good meat by throwing it away and it is cheaper than only buying muscle meat.

- Cooking with bones, livers and other bits of the animal ensures you get a wide variety of nutrients and a good balance of amino acids.

If you do not have a lot of freezer space, see if you can share large or different cuts of meat with extended family members, so you can all enjoy the benefits of grass-fed beef at very cheap prices. The other benefits of dealing with your local butcher is that they are always happy to do special cuts for you, save you some livers, and they won't look at you weirdly when you ask for a bag of bones to make bone broth!

There are some wonderful initiatives popping up in all corners of the globe about embracing locally grown food. These include projects such as community-supported agriculture (CSA), local produce swap-meets and even community gardens. These are fantastic ways to get out in the community, maybe get your hands dirty, meet new people and share in locally produced foods.

Community gardens are a great way to introduce your kids to growing new vegetables and seasonal cycles, especially if you live in a city apartment with no space to grow your own vegetables. What a fun way to get your kids excited about real food and learning about where real food comes from! And I know this works because my little nephews screw up their noses at any new vegetables their mum tries to introduce to them, but if they pick them straight from Grandpop's garden while helping him work out there, they will eat anything!

Have a look in your local area—there are so many new things happening with community food projects that you can get involved in and support. As a bonus, you get to eat local, seasonal produce. Winning all round!

Hopefully I have given you some fresh ideas to get you excited to start your own journey. There are plenty of local producers to buy from and fun, community-based ways to access local products. You will be nicely surprised with how many you find when you stop going to your big supermarket for your food and start looking small and local.

CHAPTER 19

The 28-day Reset protocol

Okay, so now you know what to eat and why to eat it; you know about weekly meal planning and that going Paleo will take some commitment; and you know that keeping a DERR diary is a useful tool for monitoring any food reactions. You're now ready to go!

I am going to give you a two-week menu plan to get you started and then outline some choices for you to follow up in the last two weeks. It is about developing your own choices for what you like to eat and experimenting for yourself.

Essentially, the 28-day Reset is an elimination diet, so it is about not eating problematic foods and changing old habits. You will not be eating from the occasional treats recipes and you will not be eating any 'grey foods'!

Menu planning and non-negotiable foods

Treats should not be a part of our everyday life, so they are not included in the 28-day Reset protocol. They should only be *occasional.* Yes, I have treat recipes in the book, but don't be under any illusions; just because they are made with Paleo ingredients does NOT mean they can be consumed daily. A treat is a treat—they are not healthy staples. Have a treat knowingly, but do not try to convince yourself otherwise.

Remember, the next 28 days are all about being good to YOU! Eat good food, move daily, sleep well, have fun and get out into nature! They are the non-negotiable essentials.

The two-week menu plans are simple and basic. If you do not like one of the recipes, just have a look back at your Paleo basics outlined in Chapter 8 and choose some meat, vegetables/fruit and some good fats to make up your meal—it is that easy! There is also no such thing as a 'breakfast staple' or a 'lunch staple' because anything you have for dinner, you can have for breakfast. This ensures that you get good levels of protein and fat in every meal.

WEEK 1

	MEAL 1	MEAL 2	MEAL 3
MONDAY	Asian Mince Breakfast Omelette	Spinach and Leek Soup with a piece of meat of your choice	Steak with Spinach Cream and Roasted Tomato
TUESDAY	Leftover Asian Mince in Lettuce Cups and Spinach and Leek Soup	Leftover Steak with Spinach Cream and Roasted Tomato	White Fish Stew (minus wine)

	MEAL 1	MEAL 2	MEAL 3
WEDNESDAY	2xEgg and Mince Muffins and The Detox Juice	White Fish Stew (minus wine)	Broccoli and Chicken Salad
THURSDAY	Leftover Broccoli and Chicken Salad	Pork Patties and mixed green salad	Chicken Meatloaf and a salad
FRIDAY	Omelette	Leftover Chicken Meatloaf and a salad	Cold Prawn and Noodle Salad
SATURDAY	Sweet Potato Fritters with Avocado Salsa	Leftover Cold Prawn and Noodle Salad	The Best Steak and Chips with a salad
SUNDAY	Eggs with Bacon-wrapped Asparagus	Leftover Sweet Potato Fritters with Avocado Salsa	Salmon and Cauli Fried Rice

WEEK 2

	MEAL 1	MEAL 2	MEAL 3
MONDAY	Leftover Salmon and Cauli Fried Rice	Basic Salad Version 3	Meatballs in Bolognese Sauce
TUESDAY	Leftover Meatballs in Bolognese Sauce	Nori Rolls	Avocado Salsa and Salmon
WEDNESDAY	Leftover Avocado and Salmon	Leftover Meatballs in Bolognese Sauce	Roasted Eggplant, Cauliflower and Warm Chicken Salad
THURSDAY	Omelette	Roasted Eggplant, Cauliflower and Warm Chicken Salad	Asian Fish En Papillote and Rainbow Salad

	MEAL 1	MEAL 2	MEAL 3
FRIDAY	Chia Seed Pudding with fruit and hardboiled eggs	Leftover Asian Fish En Papillote	Slow-cooked Osso Bucco (replace the wine with bone broth)
SATURDAY	Best-ever Brussels with eggs	Leftover Slow-cooked Osso Bucco (replace the wine with bone broth)	Bun-free Burgers
SUNDAY	2xEgg and Mince Muffins and Alkalising Juice	Dukkah-crusted Chicken Thighs with Coleslaw	Butter Chicken with Cumin-spiced Cauliflower Rice

After week 2, your meals can consist of any of the following or you can start making up your own!

WEEKS 3 AND 4

Asian Fish En Papillote

Asian Mince Breakfast Omelette

Asian Mince in Lettuce Cups

Asian-style Cabbage Salad

Asparagus, Zucchini and Roast Tomato Warm Salad

Avocado Salsa

Avocado Salsa and Salmon

Best-ever Brussels

Broccoli and Chicken Salad

Bun-free Burgers

Butter Chicken

Carrot and Sweet Potato Bites

Cashew-encrusted Lamb Chops

Cauliflower and Sweet Potato Soup

Cauliflower Bites

Chia Seed Pudding

Chicken Meatloaf

Chicken Poached in Stock with Kelp Noodles

Chicken Stuffed with Basil Pesto and Semi-sundried Tomatoes

Coconut and Turmeric Chicken Skewers

Cold Prawn and Noodle Salad

Cucumber Salad with Vietnamese Herbs

Cumin-spiced Cauliflower Rice

Coleslaw

Egg and Mince Muffins

Flax and Pumpkin Seed Crackers

Dukkah-crusted Chicken Thighs

Grilled Peach, Walnut and Beetroot Salad

Herb and Chilli Chicken

Lola's Fresh Sardine Salad

Mackerel Plaki

Meatballs in Bolognese Sauce

Nori Rolls

Omelette

Paleo Pizza

Pork Patties

Pork or Beef Lemongrass Skewers

Prawn Laksa

Radish Salad

Rainbow Salad

Roasted Eggplant, Cauliflower and Warm Chicken Salad

Salmon and Cauli Fried Rice

Slow-cooked Osso Bucco

Steak with Spinach Cream and Roasted Tomatoes

Sweet Potato Fritters

Spinach and Leek Soup

The Best Steak and Chips

218

Sweet Potato Salad

Drinks

Stick to water, coconut water, lime and soda water, and kombucha. Smoothies and juices are only to be consumed if they have been made from the recipes in this book and are not to be used as a meal replacement—they are not meals.

Snacks

Should you want to have a snack, hard-boiled eggs, activated nuts or seeds, or parsnip chips are all good options. Just make sure you are only having a small amount and it is an occasional thing. You should not feel the need to snack constantly. If you are, reassess your meal sizes and increase them.

Daily rituals

- Begin the day with a squeeze of lemon in 1/4 cup warm water. This helps to get the liver working and aids digestion.

- If you feel that you have sluggish digestion, have 1/2 teaspoon apple cider vinegar in 1/2 cup water 20 minutes before meals.

- Remember to fill in your DERR diary and make time for moving, playing and getting out into nature.

- Eat three meals per day. Do not skip any meals—eating breakfast is essential.

- Drink at least 1/2 cup bone broth daily. Bone broth is jam packed with gut-healing nutrients like glycine.

- Keep your water intake to at least 2 litres per day. This ensures you are hydrated and assists with flushing out toxins.

- Make sure you are getting at least 2 large handfuls of dark leafy greens per day. You can also include some green juices (see recipes).

Supplement considerations

As I have said before, I am a big believer in using food as medicine; however, supplements have their place. You may want to consider using some specialised supplements over the 28-day Reset protocol to give you an added boost during your program. Never start taking any new supplements without first consulting your primary healthcare practitioner.

Cod liver oil

This is a great functional food to add to your diet. It will give you good levels of EPA/DHA and additional vitamins A and D. Vitamin D is essential for production of all your hormones. Fish oils can thin the blood and are not advised if you are on blood-thinning medication or if you have clotting issues.

Magnesium

This essential mineral is involved in nearly every bodily function, and it especially gets chewed up by stress. I see magnesium deficiency a lot with my clients. Adequate levels of magnesium are essential for the absorption and metabolism of calcium and vitamin D. Look for magnesium citrate because it's a bio-available form of magnesium. It is also great for relaxing the muscles and helps you to sleep better. The recommended daily allowance (RDA) for adults is 350mg/day.

Probiotics

If you have never taken probiotics before, introduce them slowly into your eating plan using food sources first. Start with 1 tablespoon sauerkraut or 1 cup kombucha every second day, for a week. It is not recommended to start probiotic foods if you are pregnant and have never consumed them before. If you do not encounter any gastrointestinal upset, increase to daily use. If you are going to take a probiotic supplement, look for one that has multi-strains and contains micro-organisms in the billions per capsule. Take the dosage as recommended on the bottle and it is generally best taken on an empty stomach.

Frequently asked 28-day Reset questions

Can I drink coffee and tea?

Caffeine does cause a stress response in the body (cortisol release), so it should be consumed in moderation (a maximum of 1–2 cups per day). Any caffeine drinks should be consumed before lunch so as not to disturb your sleep. Assess with your DERR diary if you are using the caffeine for an energy boost, or you have excess cortisol issues—if you have, these problems need to be addressed.

Can I drink alcohol?

No. Alcohol can promote leaky gut.

What if I slip up?

Plan not to, but if you do, tomorrow is a new day. Show yourself some kindness and forgive yourself, but do not give up. Just start the next day fresh. Have a look through your DERR diary and see if you can pinpoint *why* it happened and look at addressing the issue. Was it due to stress? Was it due to not being organised? Was it due to not eating enough? Remember to always seek out the root cause of the issue.

Can I drink fruit juices?

Only if they are from recipes in this book! Fruit juices have far too much sugar and all of the goodness of the fibre taken out—you get nothing much from them other than a blood-sugar spike followed by a crash. The juice recipes you will see in the book are comprised mostly of green vegetables and non-sugary fruits such as limes.

What do I do if I have cravings?

It is understandable to have cravings, especially if you are used to eating a lot of sugar. It is a natural process that you will just need to work through, and yes, it may be a little hard, but hang in there because it won't be forever. I promise you will get over them! Cravings can usually be managed by eating something that is predominantly made up of fats or protein. My coconut cubes work a treat and so does a hard-boiled egg or chicken. Have these foods available and ready to use if you need them.

What if I am still getting gastrointestinal upsets?

Have a look and see if you have introduced too many probiotic foods too quickly or you have issues digesting FODMAPs (covered in Chapter 13). Limit these foods for a while and see how you go. Also make sure you are having your daily digestive booster of apple cider vinegar and water before meals. If you are still having issues, seek advice from a professional to help you troubleshoot the problem.

Some of your salad dressing recipes have sweeteners in them—is that okay?

This is where I tend to look at the big picture. If you have made the dressing and it has 1 teaspoon sweetener in it and that dressing will last for you eight salads, how much sugar are you really getting out of it? You still want the flavours balanced in the dressing. The key is you are not meant to completely submerge your salad in dressing. A light drizzle is all that is required. If you think after studying your DERR diary that the dressings are an issue for you, have plain salads.

I've got a headache—is that normal?

It is quite common to get a headache or two in the first few weeks of detoxing. Potentially you have cut out a lot of rubbish from your diet and your body is just having a little tantrum!

Other common 'detox' symptoms can include: acne, stuffy nose, tiredness, being emotional, poor sleep and itchy skin. These should, however, clear up over the first week or two. If you feel like something is not quite right or you are not feeling well, see your healthcare practitioner.

CHAPTER 20

Reintroducing foods

Congratulations! You've finished the 28-day Reset protocol, so now what? If you feel like you still have a way to go before you have healed your gut or sorted out some other issues, you might want to try another 28 days. If not and you are feeling good, proceed to this next phase.

Now is the time to reintroduce some of those n=1 foods (grey foods) and create your own version of Paleo. There are many ways of reintroducing foods into your diet, but I am going to share with you the way that I have found works best with my clients.

Firstly, the main thing to remember here is to only introduce one food at a time (not a food group), go slowly with it and keep your DERR diary going. This is where you will find the diary most useful. For me, there is nothing worse than watching someone be so good and complete an elimination diet and then eat a whole bunch of foods, have a reaction and then not know which food they reacted to! They need to start from scratch again! So, take it slow. Start with dairy:

- Introduce cream and butter first. Start with a small amount on the first day and then increase the amounts you consume over the course of the next three days. If you suffer no adverse reactions to these, keep them in your diet for a full seven days before adding anything else. Next try fermented dairy, such as kefir. If you are not going to eat fermented dairy, move on to probiotic dairy, such as full-fat yoghurt. Finally move on to cheese and milk. Continue adding one food over the period of a week. Add nothing else just yet. If you do react, take the foods out again and do a week of the 28-day Reset and eat cleanly for the week.

Next up are legumes:

- Make sure they are properly prepared. Again, start with small amounts of a single type of legume on the first day and slowly increase the amount you eat over the course of the week.

Next, introduce pseudo-grains:

- Same deal; test them out one at a time over the period of a week.

Time to reintroduce some of those n=1 foods (grey foods) and create your own version of Paleo.

Continue this with any other foods you may want to add back into your diet. My rule of thumb is to increase the new food over a week and then eat it for another full week before fully deciding that it agrees with you. At any point if you react to a food, go back to eating a clean 28-day Reset diet for a full week before trying another food.

To infinity and beyond!

So, what about taking Paleo into the future? You deserve congratulations for taking this journey to better your health! But now it is about continuing that success. Remember that it is a journey with lots of winding roads and it's a journey that keeps going.

If you are having issues, again remember to seek out the root cause. Keep an open mind and keep learning—this is how you will stay healthy. If you want go back to enjoying the occasional treat, do so. Just make sure that you enjoy it as a treat and don't pretend that it is a new health food. Anyway, you still need to try out some of the treats I have created in the recipe section! Have the odd glass of wine or cider with your friends. Life is there to be enjoyed!

Above all, have fun and be happy. Make the time to eat good food. Stick your feet in the dirt regularly and make bedtime your favourite time of the day (because you know how good it is for you). Hug your nearest and dearest and live life to its fullest.

CHAPTER 21

Frequently asked questions

Can I follow the Paleo template without doing the 28-day Reset protocol?

Yes you can, although it makes it harder to work out your ideal 'individual Paleo' template because you will never really know if you have any food sensitivities if you don't start with a clean slate first by doing the 28-day Reset.

Can I 'prepare' before going full-on into the 28-dayReset protocol?

Yes! Sometimes I find it easier to make gradual changes with clients before doing a 28day Reset protocol. This can help ease the detox symptoms if you have had a particularly bad diet before. What I do with some clients is:

- Slowly reduce their caffeine intake over a few weeks.

- Swap full-sugar soft drinks to lime and soda with a tablespoon of sugar, then reduce this sugar to

1 teaspoon and then no sugar over the course of a few weeks.

- Start eating three solid meals a day and reduce sugary snacks.

These small changes over a few weeks will make it much easier to do the 28-day Reset protocol when the time comes.

Will I get enough calcium following the Paleo template?

Greens such as kale and broccoli actually trump dairy for being in a form your body loves to absorb. Almonds, sunflower seeds and sesame seeds are also good choices for nondairy calcium. Another is bone broth—a Paleo staple. You do not have to consume dairy in order to get your recommended daily intake of calcium.

Can I drink alcohol?

If you are having gut issues or suspect you have leaky gut, I would say no, as alcohol can promote leaky gut. If your gut health is in order, I subscribe to the 'occasional' rule. As a general guideline, I tell my clients that the better choices are white or red wine (preservative-free, if possible), cider (reduced sugar) or tequila. Stay away from beer and other drinks that may contain gluten. My personal favourite is the Robb Wolf 'NorCal Margarita', which is tequila, fresh lime juice and soda water.

Should I get any blood tests done before starting?

I think it is worthwhile knowing where your cholesterol and triglyceride levels are at, so you can see your progress. It is also worth noting your blood pressure. A lot of people I see actually have high blood pressure and don't realise it.

What will I eat if I am not eating toast or cereal for breakfast?

You will notice in the recipe section I have recipes in the categories of Snacks, Salads, Light Meals and Larger Meals. This will be your new way of eating. There is no such thing as a 'breakfast staple' because anything you have for dinner, you can have for breakfast! This ensures that you get good levels of protein and fat (not just carbs as you do with toast and cereal) and it gives you long lasting, sustained energy throughout the day.

Am I going to lose weight following this way of eating?

If you need to balance out your weight, then yes, chances are you will lose some weight. BUT, you need to make sure that your hormones are balanced, your stress is under control, you are regularly moving and you are also sleeping well. Weight loss does not just come from changing your eating habits. If you have plateaued or are not losing weight and you have done the above to the best of your ability, seek out some expert advice from a health professional.

Without eating grains, how will I get enough fibre?

In Chapter 12 I included this table:

AVERAGE CONSUMPTION PER DAY OF FRUIT AND VEGETABLES ON A PALEO TEMPLATE

FRUIT AND VEGETABLES	FIBRE
1 cup cooked broccoli	5.2g
1/2 cup diced avocado	6g
1 cup cooked asparagus	3.6g
1 cup cooked cauliflower	2.8g
1 cucumber	1.5g
2 cups raw spinach	2g
1 cup raspberries	8g
1 cup cooked kale	3g
Total	32.1g

The total of 32.1g fibre is higher than the recommended daily intake of fibre for adults. If you are eating a proper Paleo template and eating LOADS of fresh vegetables and fruit, you will never have an issue getting enough fibre in your diet.

While we are on this subject, let's talk about poo—nutritionists love talking about poo! Why? Because it is the best indication of what is going on 'inside'. The Bristol Stool Chart shows you seven 'types' of poo ranging from hard pellet-like specimens through to watery liquid. You want to always aim for the middle ground—a nice medium-brown, smooth, soft sausage- or snake-like poo. That is a sign of good digestion and that your body likes what you are putting in there! You also want it to sink—a floating poo could be a sign of either over consumption of fats or that your gall bladder is having issues.

Will eating this way cost more?

It will, but it does not have to be monumental and there are smart things you can do to reduce your costs. Growing real food comes at a cost! When prices are always being reduced at the supermarket, someone is paying the price and it is usually the farmer. Nothing good in this life is free and we need to respect and pay reasonable prices to allow these people to have a real income.

What you can do is bypass the supermarket and head to the growers' markets and pay the farmer direct. That way, you know you are helping them out first-hand.

Buying meat in bulk is also cheaper. When we buy a half or quarter cow we are paying on average $8 per kilo! You can't even get chuck steak for that price at the supermarket and what we get for that price is all grass-fed, organic, top quality cuts of meat.

The last thing you need to remember is that you pay for convenience. You pay the same price for two chicken breasts at the supermarket as you do for a whole chicken at the market. So, what do I do? I cut up a chicken! Every time we need chicken for a recipe, I buy a whole chicken. I then cut it up and freeze the chicken wings, Marylands (entire leg of thigh and drumstick) or breasts. I wait until I have at least twelve wings in the freezer and I then take them out and bake a tray of sticky chicken wings. Don't pay someone else to cut up a chicken for you!

If I am eating out, what are the best choices for takeaway?

You have a couple of options here, provided you do not have too many sensitivities: you could take a 'Paleo leave-pass' and just enjoy whatever is on the menu or you could also make some Paleo savvy choices for meals.

It is actually not hard to eat Paleo out. Steak, anyone? A simple steak and salad with the dressing on the side is an easy option and found on most menus.

Vietnamese is another easy option. They have plenty of fresh salads, which you can combine with a protein source.

An Italian restaurant could possibly even have gluten-free pasta on the menu. Lots of restaurants understand that people have different requirements when dining out now. Much like how you can always find a vegetarian option on the menu.

If you are very sensitive to gluten, watch out for hidden sources of flour that chefs tend to put into sauces to thicken them or coat meat before cooking. A classic example of this is osso bucco. The meat is always traditionally coated in flour before browning in a pan, *before* it is slow cooked.

Always ask about the food and be very specific with your questions. If it is a good restaurant and good wait staff, they will know the answers and will be happy to assist you.

What if I am still not feeling the best after a month?

Most people start to feel a lot better after a month of eating this way. If you aren't, check your DERR diary and start to troubleshoot. What I see most often is that people are actually not eating enough. Too little fat is another common issue. I would also suggest seeking out the advice of a professional.

If I can't tolerate dairy butter can I have ghee?

Ghee is butter, but it is clarified butter. This means that it has had the milk proteins removed and you are left with just the butter fat. It is the small amount of proteins in the butter that can still upset people who are really sensitive to dairy. Most people can tolerate ghee, even if they are sensitive to butter.

You can use ghee the same way you use butter and you are able to interchange them in all of my recipes.

Why have you used coconut sugar?

Coconut sugar is a traditional sweetener used in Asian cuisine (also called palm sugar). Coconut sugar is still a processed form of sugar. I use it mainly in my desserts and occasional treats. An occasional treat is meant to be exactly that—occasional. Just because a dessert contains coconut sugar doesn't mean it is super healthy, and you should not be eating them all the time or even every week! Coconut sugar is low GI and has minerals such as magnesium, zinc and B vitamins, so it is better for you than white sugar. That is why I use it. You could always swap the coconut sugar for maple syrup, but it's still a sugar and should be used sparingly.

Why do you use pink Himalayan salt?

Pink Himalayan salt contains a full spectrum of trace minerals such as magnesium, calcium, iodine and iron and is still in its unrefined form.

Why do you say no seed oils?

The balance of omega-6 to omega-3 in today's Western diet is heavily weighted towards the six, big time! Having excess omega-6 results in stiff cell membranes, reduced cell communication, limited nutrients entering the cells and chronic inflammation.

Omegas-6s are found in seeds, nuts, grains and legumes, but where we consume it in the largest amount is through vegetable and seed oils, like soybean and canola oil. The United States saw a 5.5-fold increase in canola oil use from 1985 to 1994 and it is the third most consumed oil in the world, with soybean oil leading the way. Seed oils are just plain bad news and they should be limited in your diet as much as possible. The main culprits are soybean oil, canola oil, safflower oil and corn oil. That is why I say no seed oils.

part 2

Paleo Recipes

Condiments and Paleo essentials

Almond Milk

MAKES 3 CUPS

- 1 cup almonds, soaked overnight, drained and rinsed

- 3 cups filtered water

- 1/2 teaspoon vanilla bean paste (see Ingredients Glossary)

- pinch of pink Himalayan salt (see Ingredients Glossary)

Place all the ingredients in a blender and mix until well combined. Strain the almond milk into a jug with a lid that seals, using a nut milk bag or muslin cloth. Store in the fridge and use within 3–4 days.

Making your own almond milk is super easy. I tend to use it for cooking and only drink the occasional glass. You can keep the leftover pulp and use it in baking, wherever you see 'almond meal'.

Basil Pesto

MAKES ABOUT 1 CUP

- 1/2 cup activated cashews (see Ingredients Glossary)

- 6 marinated artichoke pieces (seed oil free) (see Ingredients Glossary)

- 3 tablespoons olive oil

- 1 large handful of basil leaves

- 1/2 long red chilli, seeded

- 1 clove garlic

- pinch of pink Himalayan salt (see Ingredients Glossary)

- freshly ground black pepper, to taste

Purée all of the ingredients together in a food processor or blender, adding more oil if required. This pesto is best eaten fresh.

I just love the addition of marinated artichoke to this pesto; it adds a different dimension to the flavour. Just make sure you read the label of the artichoke carefully and get one that is not made with seed oils, or marinate your own.

Basic Mayonnaise

MAKES ABOUT 1 CUP

- 1 egg

- 1/4 teaspoon mustard powder

- 1 teaspoon apple cider vinegar (or juice of 1/2 lemon)

- up to 3/4 cup olive oil

Whisk the egg, mustard powder and apple cider vinegar together in a small mixing bowl. Add a small stream of olive oil continuously while whisking, until the mixture is combined and the right thickness for mayonnaise (be careful not to put in too much olive oil, otherwise this will cause the mayonnaise to split). Transfer to an airtight container and store in the fridge. Use as required. The mayonnaise will last up to 7 days in the fridge.

This is my basic mayo recipe to which I add various flavours. It's a real staple in our house.

Note: Use a glass or ceramic bowl to make the mayonnaise, as lemon juice (if using) can react with a metal bowl, causing the mayonnaise to taste slightly bitter.

Horseradish Mayonnaise

MAKES ABOUT 1/3 CUP

- 4 tablespoons Basic Mayonnaise

- 1 teaspoon horseradish cream or 1 teaspoon horseradish, grated (see Ingredients Glossary)

- pink Himalayan salt, to taste (see Ingredients Glossary)

- freshly ground black pepper, to taste

Place all the ingredients in a bowl and stir until well combined. Transfer to an airtight container and store in the fridge. Use as required.

This mayonnaise goes really well with pork patties and burgers.

Dill Mayonnaise

MAKES ABOUT 1 CUP

- 1 quantity of Basic Mayonnaise

- 1 handful of dill, finely chopped

- large pinch of freshly ground black pepper

Place all the ingredients in a small bowl and stir until well combined. Transfer to an airtight container and store in the fridge. Use as required.

Garlic Aioli Mayonnaise

MAKES ABOUT 1 CUP

- 1 quantity of Basic Mayonnaise

- 1 clove garlic, minced

- large pinch of finely chopped flat-leaf (Italian) parsley

- freshly ground black pepper, to taste

Mix all the ingredients together in a bowl. Transfer to an airtight container and store in the fridge. Use as required.

Dijon Mustard Mayonnaise

MAKES ABOUT 1/3 CUP

- 3 tablespoons Basic Mayonnaise

- 1 tablespoon Dijon mustard

- 1 teaspoon raw honey (see Ingredients Glossary)

Place all the ingredients in a small bowl and stir until well combined. Transfer to an airtight container and store in the fridge. Use as required.

Sesame and Lime Dressing

MAKES ABOUT 1/3 CUP

- juice of 1 lime

- 1 long red chilli, seeded and finely chopped

- a few drops of sesame oil

- 1 teaspoon raw honey (see Ingredients Glossary)

- 2 tablespoons olive oil

- 1 teaspoon fish sauce

Place all the ingredients in a jar and shake well to combine. Drizzle over your favourite salad and enjoy!

Vietnamese Salad Dressing

MAKES ABOUT 1 1/4 CUPS

- 3 tablespoons apple cider vinegar

- 3 tablespoons fish sauce

- 1 tablespoon raw honey (see Ingredients Glossary)

- 3 cloves garlic, finely chopped

- 1 long red chilli, seeded and finely chopped

- 2/3 cup boiling water

- juice of 1 lime

Place all the ingredients in a jar and shake until well combined. Allow the flavours to infuse before serving. Store in the fridge and use as required.

> I must admit, I think if you look in my fridge at any given time, you will see this dressing. It's one of my 'go to' favourites.

Red Wine Vinaigrette

MAKES ABOUT 1/2 CUP

- 2 cloves garlic, minced

- juice of 1/2 lime

- 1 tablespoon red wine vinegar

- 3 tablespoons olive oil

- 1/4 teaspoon pink Himalayan salt (see Ingredients Glossary)

- 1/2 teaspoon freshly ground black pepper

Combine all the ingredients in a bowl and allow the flavours to develop for 5–10 minutes before serving.

> This vinaigrette works well drizzled over a green salad or even on top of freshly shucked oysters.

Curry Salad Dressing

MAKES ABOUT 1/3 CUP

- 2 tablespoons apple cider vinegar
- 1 teaspoon raw honey (see Ingredients Glossary)
- 1 teaspoon wholegrain mustard
- 1/2 teaspoon curry powder
- 2 tablespoons olive oil

Place all of the ingredients in a jar and shake well to combine. Store in the fridge and use as required.

> Apple cider vinegar in dressings is a great way to help improve your digestion, as it increases digestive secretions.

Honey Wholegrain Mustard Dressing

MAKES ABOUT 1/2 CUP

- 1 tablespoon wholegrain mustard
- 1 teaspoon raw honey (see Ingredients Glossary)

- juice of 1/2 lemon

- 3 tablespoons olive oil

Place all the ingredients in a jar and shake well to combine. Store in the fridge and use as required.

> I love salads and salad dressings! The trick is to not overdress them; salads only need a hint of dressing.

Blueberry Balsamic Reduction

MAKES 1/4 CUP

- 3/4 cup balsamic vinegar

- 1 tablespoon raw honey (see Ingredients Glossary)

- 1 cup blueberries

Place all the ingredients into a small saucepan and bring to the boil. Simmer, uncovered, until the mixture thickens, then strain and discard the blueberries. Store the reduction in a sealed glass jar in the fridge.

> I drizzle this wonderful reduction over my favourite salad combinations. It works particularly well with salads that have fruits in them, providing a lovely balance of sweet and slightly sour.

Tomato Sauce

MAKES 2 CUPS

- 2 teaspoons apple cider vinegar

- 1x400g (14oz) tin whole tomatoes

- freshly ground black pepper, to taste

- 1 tablespoon raw honey (see Ingredients Glossary)

- pinch of ground cloves

- 2 teaspoons sambal (see Ingredients Glossary)

- 3 tablespoons tomato paste

Place all the ingredients in a food processor or blender and mix until well combined. Transfer to a sealable glass jar and refrigerate. Use as required. The sauce will last for a couple of weeks in the fridge.

> Every house needs a good tomato sauce in the fridge. So why not have one that you KNOW does not have any added salt, sugar or hidden nasties in it?

Sweet Chilli Sauce

MAKES ABOUT 1/2 CUP

- 1/3 cup coconut sugar (see Ingredients Glossary)

- 1/2 cup apple cider vinegar

- 1 long red chilli, seeded and finely chopped

- 3 medjool dates, pitted and finely chopped (see Ingredients Glossary)

Put the coconut sugar, apple cider vinegar, chilli and dates in a small saucepan over a medium heat and bring to the boil, stirring continuously. Reduce the heat and simmer, stirring continuously, until the mixture thickens. Allow to cool, then store in a jar or glass bottle in the fridge. Use as required.

> This has a nice sweet and sour flavour with a hot kick to it! Yes, this does have some coconut sugar in it, but you don't use much of this sauce in recipes, so it's not worth stressing about. If you don't want to use the coconut sugar, use 9 medjool dates in total instead.

Red Wine and Peppercorn Sauce

MAKES ABOUT 1/2 CUP

- 3 tablespoons butter or ghee (see Ingredients Glossary)

- 1/2 red (Spanish) onion, minced

- 1 clove garlic, minced

- 2 tablespoons green peppercorns, crushed

- 1/2 cup good red wine

- 1 tablespoon balsamic vinegar

- 1 small handful of flat-leaf (Italian) parsley, finely chopped

Heat 2 tablespoons of the butter in a pan over a medium heat. Add the onion and garlic and sauté until translucent and soft. Add the peppercorns and cook for a further 30 seconds, then add the wine and balsamic vinegar and bring to the boil. Simmer until the liquid has reduced by half, then add the final tablespoon of butter and stir through. Spoon the sauce on top of your chosen meat, sprinkle over the parsley and serve.

> This is a full-flavoured sauce that works well with kangaroo, other game meats or any dark meats.

Avocado Salsa

SERVES 2, OR 4–6 AS PART OF A MEAL

- 1/2 red capsicum (pepper), diced

- 1/2 green capsicum (pepper), diced

- 1/2 yellow capsicum (pepper), diced

- 10 grape tomatoes, quartered

- 1 handful of baby spinach leaves, roughly chopped

- 1 small handful of flat-leaf (Italian) parsley, finely chopped

- 1 small handful of coriander (cilantro), finely chopped

- 1 spring onion (scallion), finely chopped

- 1/2 long red chilli, seeded and finely chopped

- pinch of pink Himalayan salt (see Ingredients Glossary)

- freshly ground black pepper, to taste

- 1 clove garlic, minced

- 1 small avocado, diced

- extra virgin olive oil, for drizzling

Mix all the ingredients, except the olive oil, together in a large bowl then drizzle with the oil and allow to sit for 10 minutes so the flavours infuse.

This salsa is jam packed with nutrients, as you can see by all the bright colours in the dish. The addition of avocado gives you a good dose of heart-healthy monounsaturated fats.

Bolognese Sauce

SERVES 8–10

- 1 tablespoon butter
- 1 brown onion, roughly chopped
- 2 cloves garlic, roughly chopped
- 1/2 small butternut pumpkin, roughly chopped
- 3 sticks celery, roughly chopped
- 1 small sweet potato (kumara), peeled and roughly chopped
- 1 large carrot, roughly chopped
- 1 small zucchini (courgette), roughly chopped
- 1 long red chilli, seeded, finely chopped
- 2x400g (14oz) tins whole tomatoes
- 2 large tomatoes, quartered
- 3 tablespoons tomato paste
- 1/2 teaspoon ground paprika
- 1 teaspoon dried basil
- 1 teaspoon freshly ground black pepper
- 2 cups Bone Broth (see recipe opposite) or beef stock

Melt the butter in a large heavy-based pot over a medium heat. Add the onion and garlic and sauté until soft. Add the pumpkin, celery, sweet potato and carrot, stirring for 3–5 minutes, then add the zucchini, chilli, tinned tomatoes, fresh tomatoes, tomato paste, paprika, basil and pepper, stirring for another 2 minutes. Add the bone broth and simmer, covered, for 15 minutes, or until the vegetables are soft. Remove the pot from the heat and blend the mixture to a smooth consistency using a hand blender. Adjust the seasoning and serve.

This Bolognese sauce is very versatile and you can use it in many dishes. It is packed with vegetables and has the gut-healing power of the Bone Broth. It's an easy way to get vegetables into fussy eaters.

Tip: Add additional Bone Broth if you want a thinner sauce. I never add salt to this sauce as I find that the minerals from the Bone Broth give it enough flavour. Test the flavour yourself and add salt to taste if you desire.

Bone Broth

MAKES ABOUT 8 CUPS

- 1 tablespoon butter
- 1/2 brown onion, roughly chopped

- 3 cloves garlic, roughly chopped

- 2 sticks celery, roughly chopped

- 1 large carrot, roughly chopped

- 3 tablespoons apple cider vinegar

- 1 tablespoon black whole peppercorns

- 2–3kg (4lb 8oz–6lb 12oz) beef bones with marrow

Heat the butter in a large pot over a medium heat. Add the onion and garlic and cook until fragrant and soft. Add the celery and carrot, cooking for a further 5 minutes, then add the apple cider vinegar, peppercorns, bones and enough water to completely submerge the bones. Bring to the boil, then simmer, covered, for anywhere from 24 to 72 hours. Add more water as required to keep the bones covered. After cooking, the bones should be brittle and crumbly.

Remove any larger bone from the broth with tongs and strain the remaining liquid. Place the broth in the fridge to cool overnight so that a top layer of fat forms.

The next day, scrape this top layer off and discard. The remaining cold broth should be of a gelatinous consistency.

Divide the broth into 2-cup portions and freeze or store in the fridge. Use as required.

Bone broth is rich, full of nutrients and wonderfully healing. It is great to get in the habit of making a big batch on the weekends and having some every day (about 1/2 cup). You will feel the benefits, I promise! It is also a great way to get some additional calcium into your diet.

Tip: Some recipes say to simmer for as little as 12 hours but I feel that a minimum of 24 hours is required to get the best release of nutrients and minerals from the bones—the longer, the better.

Love Your Greens Dip

MAKES ABOUT 1 CUP

- 3 handfuls of basil leaves

- 1 small avocado, halved

- 1 clove garlic

- 3 tablespoons olive oil

- 1 handful of baby spinach leaves, stems trimmed

- 4 marinated artichoke pieces (seed oil free) (see Ingredients Glossary)

- 1 teaspoon apple cider vinegar

- pink Himalayan salt, to taste (see Ingredients Glossary)

- freshly ground black pepper, to taste

Place all the ingredients in a food processor or blender and mix until puréed. Transfer to an airtight container and store in the fridge. Use as required.

Serve with Flax and Pumpkin Seed Crackers (see recipe on below pages) or raw vegetable sticks.

> A sneaky way to get the family to eat a whole bunch of greens!

Hot Salsa

SERVES 4–6 AS PART OF A MEAL

- 1 tablespoon butter
- 1 brown onion, diced
- 1 long red chilli, seeded and finely chopped
- 3 cloves garlic, finely chopped
- 1/2 teaspoon ground turmeric
- 1/2 teaspoon ground paprika
- 1/2 teaspoon ground coriander
- 1/2 teaspoon ground cumin
- 3 whole tomatoes, diced
- 1 medium zucchini (courgette), finely chopped

- 6 cauliflower florets, finely chopped

- 1 red capsicum (pepper), finely chopped

- 1 large carrot, finely chopped

- 1x400g (14oz) tin whole tomatoes

- 2 tablespoons tomato paste

- 3/4 cup vegetable stock

- 1 handful of coriander (cilantro), roughly chopped

- freshly ground black pepper, to taste

Melt the butter in a pan over a medium heat. Add the onion, chilli and garlic and cook until soft. Add the turmeric, paprika, coriander and cumin and cook, stirring continuously, until fragrant. Add the tomatoes, zucchini, cauliflower, capsicum, carrot, tinned tomatoes, tomato paste and vegetable stock and stir to combine. Bring to the boil, then simmer, uncovered, for 20 minutes or until the vegetables are soft and the sauce has thickened. Stir through the coriander leaves and season with the pepper. Allow the mixture to cool then transfer to an airtight container and store in the fridge.

This salsa is spicy hot—just how I like it! You can always ease off on the chilli if you don't want it so hot. It is great served over steamed vegetables as part of a meal or with crackers and veggie sticks as a dip. It is also full of antioxidant compounds such as lycopene from all the cooked tomatoes.

Note: Use as a dip or serve over salmon steaks, topped with activated macadamia nuts and coriander leaves as a meal.

Lacto-fermented Sauerkraut

MAKES ABOUT 2X1-LITRE JARS

- 1 medium red cabbage, shredded (keep 2 outer leaves)

- 1 medium white cabbage, shredded

- 2 carrots, grated

- 2 tablespoons pink Himalayan salt (see Ingredients Glossary)

- 2 large glass jars (at least 1 litre each) with sealed lids

Toss the red and white cabbage, carrot and salt together in a large mixing bowl and squeeze the mixture together with your hands to break up the cellular structure of the vegetables (this takes a bit of elbow grease).

When the mixture has become limp and a lot of juice has been released, evenly distribute the mixture into the jars. Pack the vegetables and juice in as tightly as you can (the vegetables must be completely submerged by liquid), leaving about 2–3cm (3/4–1 1/4in) at the top.

Press the spare cabbage leaves down over the top of the mixture, making sure they keep the vegetables submerged. Cover the top of the jars loosely with muslin and allow the mixture to sit at room temperature, undisturbed, for around seven days. You can test the sauerkraut every few days, until it is done to your liking (it can stay at room temperature for up to 3–4 weeks). When done, remove the top cabbage leaves, place the proper lids on the jars and transfer to the refrigerator, where it will keep for at least 6 months.

Learning to make your own probiotic foods is one of the easiest and best ways to improve your gut health. Make eating probiotic foods a part of your day. It also helps that they taste yummy!

Dukkah Mix

MAKES ABOUT 3/4 CUP

- 125g (4 1/2oz) activated pistachios (see Ingredients Glossary)
- 1/2 teaspoon ground cumin
- 1/2 teaspoon ground coriander
- 1/2 teaspoon dried oregano

- 1/2 teaspoon dried thyme

- 1/2 teaspoon chilli flakes

- 4 tablespoons toasted sesame seeds

- pink Himalayan salt, to taste (see Ingredients Glossary)

- freshly ground black pepper, to taste

Place all the ingredients into a blender or food processor and process to a coarse powder. Store in an airtight container and use as required.

> This dukkah mix works well as a crumb for chicken, fish and lamb. It's also yummy sprinkled straight onto salads for some additional crunch.

Claire's Tasty Paleo Granola

MAKES ABOUT 12 CUPS

- 3–4 cups toasted coconut chips or flakes (not desiccated)

- 2 cups activated sunflower seeds, roughly chopped (see Ingredients Glossary)

- 1 cup activated pumpkin seeds (pepitas) (see Ingredients Glossary)

- 2 cups activated cashews, roughly chopped (see Ingredients Glossary)

- 1/2 cup activated hazelnuts, roughly chopped (see Ingredients Glossary)

- 5 medjool dates, pitted and roughly chopped (see Ingredients Glossary)

- 2 cups activated macadamia nuts, roughly chopped (see Ingredients Glossary)

- 1/2 cup activated almonds, roughly chopped (see Ingredients Glossary)

- 10 dried apricot halves, roughly chopped (sulphur free)

- 1/4 cup activated pistachios, roughly chopped (see Ingredients Glossary)

- 2 tablespoons raw honey (see Ingredients Glossary)

- 1/2 cup coconut oil

Preheat the oven to 170°C (325°F).

Line two baking trays with baking paper.

Place all the ingredients in a large bowl and mix until well combined. Spread the mixture evenly over the two baking trays and bake for 30 minutes, mixing halfway through. Remove from the oven and set aside to cool.

Store in airtight containers in the fridge and use as required.

This makes a lot of granola! But it stays perfect if stored in the fridge, so that the oils in the nuts and seeds do not go rancid. You can use it as a sprinkle on desserts or as an occasional breakfast treat.

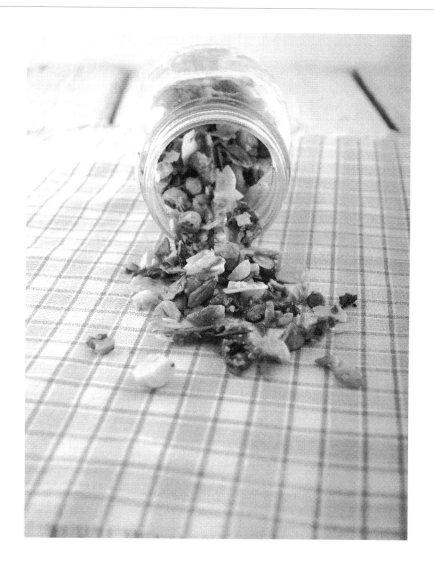

Asian Egg Crêpes

MAKES APPROXIMATELY 6

- 3 eggs

- 1 teaspoon fish sauce

- 1 teaspoon coconut aminos or tamari sauce (see Ingredients Glossary for both)

- freshly ground black pepper, to taste

- 1 teaspoon butter or ghee (see Ingredients Glossary)

Whisk the eggs, fish sauce, coconut aminos and pepper together in a bowl.

Melt the butter in a wok or frying pan, then pour one-sixth of the egg mixture into the pan while swirling until you have a thin crêpe. Flip the crêpe and cook for a further 10 seconds, then set aside and repeat with the remaining mixture. Serve immediately.

These crêpes may smell a bit strong when you make them on their own, but trust me, mixed into the Asian Mince recipe or in the Nori Rolls, they add just the right amount of flavour.

Paleo Pizza Base

MAKES 1

- 1 cup activated almonds (see Ingredients Glossary)
- 1 cup activated cashews (see Ingredients Glossary)
- 1 tablespoon dried oregano
- 5 sprigs of flat-leaf (Italian) parsley, finely chopped
- 1/4 teaspoon bicarbonate of soda
- pink Himalayan salt, to taste (see Ingredients Glossary)
- freshly ground black pepper, to taste
- 2 eggs

Preheat the oven to 180°C (350°F).

Place the almonds and cashews into a food processor or blender and pulse to a fine crumble. Stir in the oregano, parsley, bicarbonate of soda, salt and pepper, then add the eggs and continuing stirring until combined (the mixture should be quite moist).

Turn out the mixture onto a flat surface lined with baking paper and place another sheet on top (this stops it from sticking when rolling it flat). Roll out to roughly 2–3mm (1/16–1/8in) in thickness.

Lift the pizza base using the baking paper and place onto a baking or pizza tray, removing the top sheet of baking paper. Add your selected toppings and bake for approximately 15–20 minutes. Serve immediately.

Pizza does not have to be a bad word. It is what you make it with that counts! Use this recipe as your 'go to' basic base and then load it up with your favourite vegetable and meat combos. You do not have to order takeaway to enjoy pizza!

Drinks, Smoothies and Juices

Alkalising Juice

SERVES 2

- 1 large bunch of baby spinach leaves, stems trimmed

- 3 sticks celery

- 2cm (3/4in) piece of fresh ginger, peeled

- 1 lime, quartered (leave skin on)

- 1 large Lebanese cucumber

Combine all the ingredients in a juicer and consume within 24 hours.

A perfect juice to have daily, as it is packed with nutrients and antioxidants. This juice is also a great anti-ageing elixir.

The Detox Juice

SERVES 1

- 1/2 apple, cored
- 1 large handful of baby spinach leaves, stems trimmed
- 2 beetroots, including the leaves, scrubbed
- 5 sticks celery
- 2cm (3/4in) piece of fresh ginger, peeled

Combine all the ingredients in a juicer and consume within 24 hours.

> Greens are perfect for alkalising the body and aiding the detox process, and the ginger is wonderfully calming on the gut. The beetroot leaves give you a nice dose of vitamins A and C and they are also full of magnesium.

Inflammation Buster

SERVES 1

- 2cm (3/4in) piece of fresh ginger, peeled
- 1 lemon, quartered (leave skin on)

- 2cm (3/4in) piece of fresh turmeric or 1/2 teaspoon ground turmeric (see Ingredients Glossary)

- 1/2 carrot

- 1/2 green apple

- 1 cup filtered water

Combine all the ingredients in a juicer and consume within 24 hours.

Turmeric is a powerful anti-inflammatory agent. If you are having issues with inflammation, turmeric is a must-have addition to your diet. Combine it with ginger and lemon, and you are well on your way to bringing your inflammation down. The carrot and apple add some natural sweetness to the juice.

Banana Smoothie

SERVES 2

- 2 frozen ripe bananas

- 1 handful of activated macadamia nuts (see Ingredients Glossary)

- 2 tablespoons activated pumpkin seeds (pepitas) (see Ingredients Glossary)

- 1 tablespoon chia seeds (see Ingredients Glossary)

- 1 cup almond milk (see recipe on above pages)

- 1 cup filtered water

Combine all the ingredients in a blender until smooth.

I love a good banana smoothie. This one is great after a workout, and the addition of macadamia nuts gives you the added bonus of some good fats. If you don't like eating over-ripe bananas, peel and store them in the freezer to use in this smoothie later.

Chocolate and Banana Smoothie

SERVES 2

- 1 large ripe banana

- 1 tablespoon raw cacao powder (see Ingredients Glossary)

- 1 handful of activated macadamia nuts, roughly chopped, plus extra, to garnish (see Ingredients Glossary)

- 2 cups almond milk (see recipe on above pages)

- 1 small handful of cacao nibs (see Ingredients Glossary)

Place the banana, raw cacao powder, macadamia nuts and almond milk in a blender and mix until well combined. Pour into two serving glasses, then top with the cacao nibs and reserved macadamias.

Tip: You can sprinkle over some additional raw cacao powder instead of the cacao nibs.

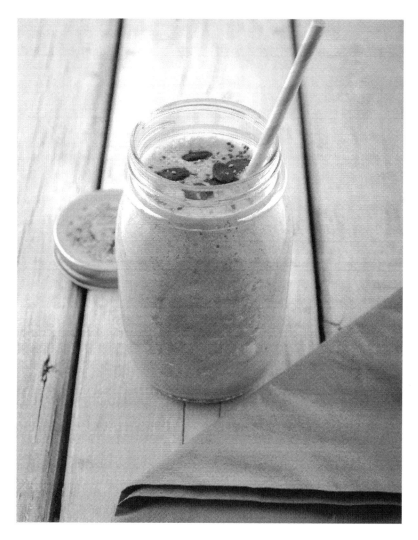

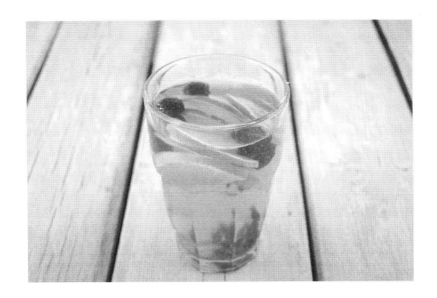

Raspberry and Lime Drink

SERVES 1

- 1 cup coconut water
- 1/2 cup raspberries
- juice of 1/2 lime
- 1/2 lime, cut into slices

Place all the ingredients into a large glass, stir gently and drink.

Chocolate Milkshake

SERVES 2

- 1 handful of baby spinach leaves, stems trimmed

- 1 handful of raspberries

- 1 cup almond milk (see recipe on above pages)

- 2 cups filtered water

- 1 tablespoon chia seeds (see Ingredients Glossary)

- 2 tablespoons raw cacao powder (see Ingredients Glossary)

Combine all the ingredients in a blender until smooth.

> Trust me, you will never taste the spinach leaves! It is a great way to sneak some additional greens into your day.

Hot Chocolate

SERVES 2

- 1/4 cup coconut milk

- 1 cup water

- 1 teaspoon raw cacao powder (see Ingredients Glossary)

- 1 tablespoon cacao butter (see Ingredients Glossary)

- 1 teaspoon coconut sugar (see Ingredients Glossary)

- pinch of pink Himalayan salt (see Ingredients Glossary)

- sprinkle of cacao nibs (see Ingredients Glossary)

Place the coconut milk, water, cacao powder, cacao butter, coconut sugar and salt in a small saucepan and gently heat (to as hot as you want) until the coconut sugar has dissolved. Pour into two mugs, sprinkle with cacao nibs and serve.

I love having this warming hot chocolate on a cold winter's night. I find that the coconut milk sweetens it enough for me and I leave out the coconut sugar. The cacao butter gives it a luxurious, creamy chocolate taste—enjoy!

Snacks, salads, light meals and sides

Activated Nut and Seed Trail Mix

MAKES ABOUT 2–3 CUPS

- 1 handful of activated macadamia nuts (see Ingredients Glossary)

- 1 handful of activated almonds (see Ingredients Glossary)

- 1 handful of activated pumpkin seeds (pepitas) (see Ingredients Glossary)

- 1 small handful of activated sunflower seeds (see Ingredients Glossary)

- 1 handful of coconut flakes (not desiccated coconut)

Mix the activated nuts and seeds with the coconut flakes and store in an airtight container in the fridge. Use as required.

This is a great mix to have in the fridge, ready to go if you need a snack.

Lime, Honey and Black Pepper Parsnip Chips

SERVES 4

- 5 large parsnips
- zest and juice of 2 small limes
- 3 tablespoons olive oil
- 2 teaspoons raw honey (see Ingredients Glossary)
- 1/2 teaspoon freshly ground black pepper

Slice the parsnips into chips using a mandolin.

Place the lime zest and juice, olive oil, raw honey and pepper in a bowl and stir until well combined. Using your hands, gently toss the parsnip chips in the oil and honey mix, making sure the chips are well coated.

If using an oven, spread the chips out onto baking trays lined with baking paper and bake at your oven's lowest temperature (70–100°C/150–200°F) with the door slightly ajar, until crisp.

If using a dehydrator, spread your chips on the trays provided and dehydrate according to the dehydrator's instructions.

> These are great, zesty and the whole family will love them—a perfect snack when watching movies!

Flax and Pumpkin Seed Crackers

MAKES 20–30

- 1 cup almond meal
- 1/2 cup flax seeds (see Ingredients Glossary)
- 1 tablespoon chia seeds (see Ingredients Glossary)
- pink Himalayan salt, to taste (see Ingredients Glossary)
- freshly ground black pepper, to taste
- 1/4 cup activated pumpkin seeds (pepitas) (see Ingredients Glossary)
- 1 egg
- 1 tablespoon coconut oil

Preheat the oven to 170°C (325°F).

Place all the ingredients in a food processor or blender and mix until a dough forms. Turn out the dough onto a flat surface lined with baking paper and place another sheet on top (this stops the dough from sticking when rolling flat). Roll the dough to roughly a 2–3mm (1/16–1/8in) thickness. Remove the top sheet of baking paper and, with a sharp knife, lightly score the top of the mixture into squares. I usually make the squares 2cmx2cm (3/4inx3/4in), but you can make them as big as you like.

Place the dough onto the tray using the baking paper and bake for 15–20 minutes until cooked through, then allow to cool on the tray.

Break up the crackers and store them in an airtight container in the fridge.

These versatile crackers keep well in the fridge. If you make the scores in them larger, you can use them as lunch crackers, topped with tuna and salad.

Smoked Salmon and Horseradish on Flax and Pumpkin Seed Crackers

MAKES 15–20

- 1/2 teaspoon fresh horseradish, grated, or 1 teaspoon horseradish cream (see Ingredients Glossary)

- 1 portion of Basic Mayonnaise (see recipe on above pages)

- 15–20 Flax and Pumpkin Seed Crackers (see recipe on above pages)

- 1 small Lebanese cucumber, sliced into rounds

- 200g (7oz) smoked salmon

- 1 small handful of dill, to garnish

- freshly ground black pepper, to taste

Place the horseradish and Basic Mayonnaise in a bowl and mix until well combined.

Lay out the crackers and add to each a round of cucumber, a dollop of horseradish mayonnaise, a little smoked salmon, a sprig of dill and a pinch of pepper. Serve immediately.

These crackers look so pretty and taste amazing—guaranteed to win everyone over at your next dinner party or BBQ!

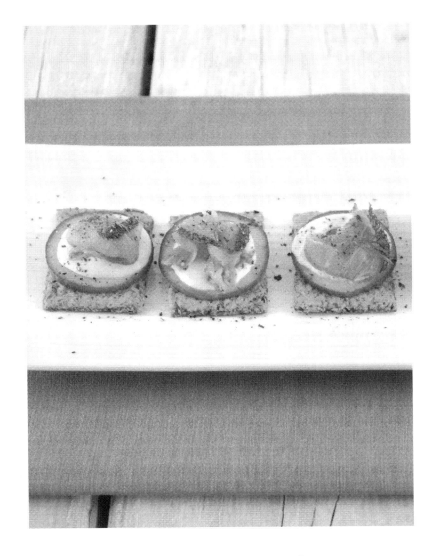

Paprika Sweet Potato Chips

SERVES 4

- 5 small sweet potatoes (kumara), peeled
- 1/2 teaspoon apple cider vinegar
- 3 teaspoons olive oil
- 2 teaspoons maple syrup

- 1/4 teaspoon ground paprika

- 1/2 teaspoon freshly ground black pepper

Slice the sweet potatoes into chips using a mandolin.

Place the apple cider vinegar, olive oil, maple syrup, paprika and pepper in a bowl and stir until well combined. Using your hands, gently toss the sweet potato chips through the oil and maple syrup mix, making sure the chips are well coated.

If using an oven, spread the chips out on baking trays lined with baking paper and bake at your oven's lowest temperature (70–100°C/150–200°F) with the door slightly ajar, until crisp.

If using a dehydrator, spread your chips on the trays provided and dehydrate according to the dehydrator's instructions.

Watch out—these chips are moreish!

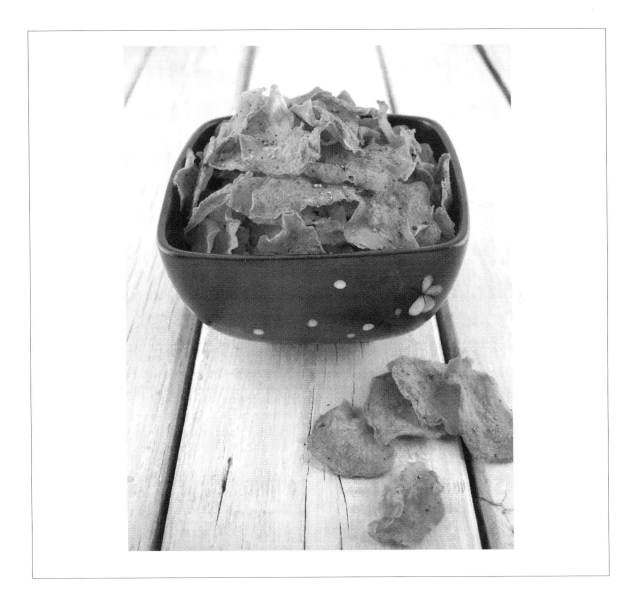

Carrot and Sweet Potato Bites

MAKES 20–24

- 1 small sweet potato (kumara), peeled and cubed
- 2 medium carrots, 1 diced and 1 grated
- 1/2 large zucchini (courgette), grated

- 3 tablespoons activated pine nuts (see Ingredients Glossary)

- 2 tablespoons activated macadamia nuts, roughly chopped (see Ingredients Glossary)

- 1 teaspoon dried chilli flakes

- 1 teaspoon ground cumin

- 3 spring onions (scallions), finely chopped

- 1 handful of coriander (cilantro), finely chopped

- 1 handful of dill, finely chopped

- 1 tablespoon raw honey (see Ingredients Glossary)

- 1 egg

- 6 tablespoons almond meal

- pink Himalayan salt, to taste (see Ingredients Glossary)

- freshly ground black pepper, to taste

- butter, ghee (see Ingredients Glossary) or coconut oil, for frying

- Dill Mayonnaise, to serve (see recipe on below pages)

Place the sweet potato and diced carrot in a steamer and steam until cooked through. Transfer to a bowl, roughly mash with a fork and set aside.

Squeeze out any excess water from the grated carrot and zucchini and place in a large mixing bowl. Add the pine nuts, macadamia nuts, chilli, cumin, spring onion, coriander and dill and stir until well combined. Mix through the honey and egg, then the almond meal—the mixture should be moist but not too wet (if it is, add a little more almond meal). Season with salt and pepper.

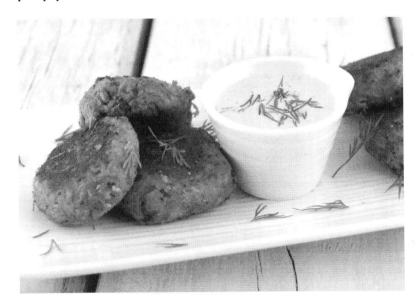

Using your hands, mould bite-sized balls out of the mixture.

Melt butter in a pan over a medium heat and fry the bites until brown all over. Serve hot or cold with the Dill Mayonnaise.

These little bites make great snacks or lunchbox treats. Just leave out the chilli if you are making them for the kids. They have a good mix of carbohydrates from the carrots and sweet potato and good fats from the nuts.

Cauliflower Bites

SERVES 4 AS A SNACK

Za'atar Mix

- 4 tablespoons sesame oil

- 4 teaspoons ground sumac (see Ingredients Glossary)

- 2 teaspoons dried thyme

- 1 teaspoon ground cumin

- 1/2 teaspoon pink Himalayan salt (see Ingredients Glossary)

- 1/2 head of cauliflower, cut into small bite-sized florets

Preheat the oven to 200°C (400°F).

Line a baking tray with baking paper.

Place the za'atar ingredients in a large bowl and, using a hand blender, mix until well combined. Gently toss the cauliflower through the za'atar mix, making sure the cauliflower is well coated.

Spread the cauliflower florets evenly around the baking tray, making sure they are spaced nicely apart. Bake in the oven for 20 minutes or until golden brown. Serve immediately.

Za'atar is a Middle Eastern spice mix that works really well with cauliflower. These little bites are moreish and make a great healthy snack.

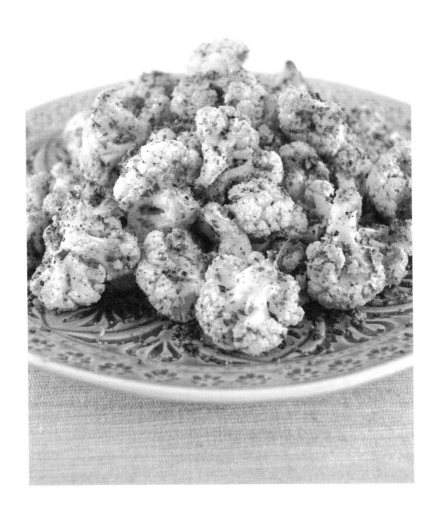

Asian-style Cabbage Salad

SERVES 4

- 1/4 white cabbage, shredded

- 1/4 red cabbage, shredded

- 2 small Lebanese cucumbers, cut into batons

- 1 large carrot, grated

- 1 spring onion (scallion), finely chopped

- 1 large handful of baby spinach leaves, roughly chopped

- 1 handful of coriander (cilantro), roughly chopped

- 1 small red capsicum (pepper), finely sliced

- drizzle of Sesame and Lime Dressing (see recipe on above pages)

- 1 tablespoon sesame seeds, to garnish

- 1 tablespoon dulse flakes, to garnish (see Ingredients Glossary)

- 1 lime, cut in wedges, to serve

Place the white and red cabbage, cucumber, carrot, spring onion, spinach, coriander and capsicum in a bowl and mix until well combined. Drizzle the Sesame and Lime Dressing over the salad, sprinkle with the sesame seeds and dulse flakes and serve with a wedge of lime.

This is another vibrant Asian-inspired salad. It works really well with any kind of fish or seafood. Leave off the dressing if you want to use the salad the next day and then add the dressing just before you eat.

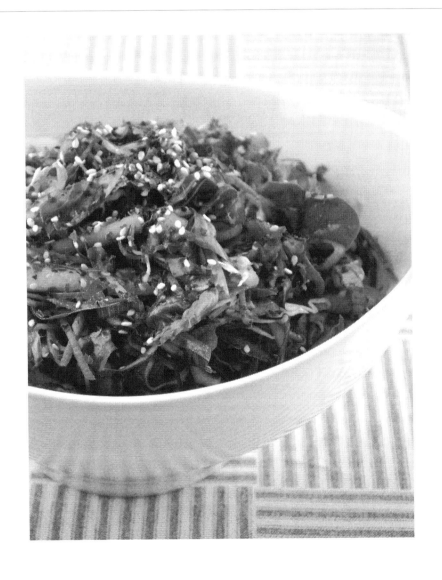

Asparagus, Zucchini and Roast Tomato Warm Salad

SERVES 2, OR 4 AS PART OF A MEAL

- 20 grape tomatoes, halved

- pink Himalayan salt, to taste (see Ingredients Glossary)

- freshly ground black pepper, to taste

- 14 asparagus spears, lower ends trimmed

- 5 baby zucchinis (courgettes), thinly sliced lengthways

- 2 slices of goat's haloumi (omit if you are sensitive to dairy or on the 28-day Reset)

- 2 tablespoons Basil Pesto (see recipe on above pages)

- 1 tablespoon activated pumpkin seeds (pepitas) (see Ingredients Glossary)

Preheat the oven to 180°C (350°F).

Place the tomatoes on a baking tray lined with baking paper. Season with salt and pepper and bake for 15–20 minutes.

While the tomatoes are baking, grill the asparagus and zucchini until tender.

Heat a griddle pan over a medium heat and grill the haloumi on both sides until golden. Set aside.

Toss the asparagus and zucchini with the Basil Pesto in a bowl, reserving a small amount of pesto to garnish.

Arrange the asparagus and zucchini on a serving platter and add the tomatoes. Crumble over the haloumi, then sprinkle with the pumpkin seeds and remaining pesto. Serve immediately.

A winner for every occasion! This is a bright and colourful dish that gets your tastebuds going as soon as you see it.

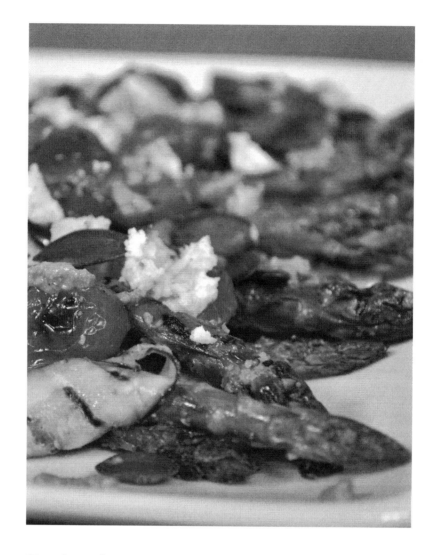

Basic Salad Four Ways

SERVES 1, OR 2 AS PART OF A MEAL

- 1 large Lebanese cucumber, diced
- 2 handfuls of baby spinach leaves, roughly chopped
- 1 handful of cherry tomatoes, halved
- 1/2 red capsicum (pepper), roughly chopped

- 1 spring onion (scallion), finely chopped

Mix all the ingredients together in a large bowl and serve.

> This basic salad mix is a standard in our house. Just make sure you always have these main vegetables in your fridge and then you can always have a quick salad ready in no time. Just add some protein and a little fat/oil and you are done—quick, healthy and simple!

Version 1
Flake 1x210g (7 1/2oz) tin of salmon over the salad. Dress with Sesame and Lime Dressing (see recipe on above pages) and serve.

Version 2
Season a chicken breast with freshly ground black pepper. Melt 1 tablespoon butter in a pan over a medium heat and cook the chicken breast until golden brown on both sides and cooked through. Slice the breast and add to the salad. Drizzle with Dijon Mustard Mayonnaise (see recipe on above pages) and serve.

Version 3
Slice 2 hard-boiled eggs and mix into the salad. Dress with the Honey Wholegrain Mustard Dressing (see recipe on above pages) and serve.

Version 4
Roughly chop a handful of macadamia nuts and mix through the salad. Sprinkle with 1 teaspoon Dukkah Mix (see recipe on above pages) and serve.

Cumin-spiced Cauliflower Rice

SERVES 4

- 2 teaspoons ghee (see Ingredients Glossary) or butter

- 2 teaspoons cumin seeds

- 1/2 large brown onion, finely chopped

- 3/4 large head of cauliflower, grated

Heat the ghee in a pan over a medium to high heat. Add the cumin seeds and cook until fragrant, then add the onion and cook until soft and translucent, stirring frequently. Add the grated cauliflower and cook for a further 2 minutes, stirring frequently.

> This cauliflower is unbelievably tasty. You would never know that it is not white rice.

Tip: Do not cook the cauliflower for too long; it should remain crisp.

Cold Prawn and Noodle Salad

SERVES 4

- 2 tablespoons apple cider vinegar
- 2 tablespoons fish sauce
- 2 tablespoons lime juice
- 2 teaspoons raw honey (see Ingredients Glossary)
- 1 long red chilli, seeded and finely chopped
- 1 large carrot, julienned
- 1/4 medium red cabbage, shredded
- 1/2 red capsicum (pepper), thinly sliced lengthways
- 1 spring onion (scallion), finely chopped
- 1 handful of mung bean shoots
- 1 handful of snow peas (mangetout), ends trimmed and cut lengthways
- 1 small handful of mint leaves, roughly torn, plus extra to serve
- 1 small handful of coriander (cilantro), roughly torn, plus extra to serve
- 1 tablespoon coconut oil
- 2 cloves garlic, crushed

- 20 medium raw prawns, peeled and deveined with tails intact

- 1x340g (11 3/4oz) packet kelp noodles (see Ingredients Glossary)

- 1 lime, quartered, to serve

First make the dressing. Place the apple cider vinegar, fish sauce, lime juice, honey and chilli in a small jar and shake until well combined. Set aside.

In a large bowl, combine the carrot, cabbage, capsicum, spring onion, mung beans and snow peas. Add the mint and coriander.

Heat the coconut oil in a pan over a medium heat. When hot, add the garlic and fry for 10 seconds. Add the prawns in two batches, cooking for about 2 minutes each side, until the prawns turn pink and are cooked through, then set aside.

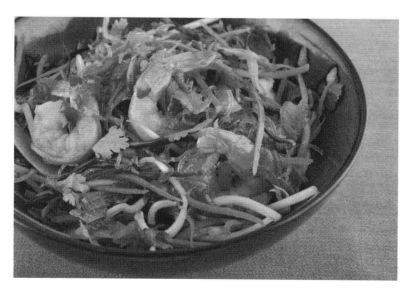

Place the noodles in a large bowl, cover them with hot water and soak for 2 minutes until the noodles are soft. Drain through a colander, making sure to separate any noodles that are clumped together. Add the noodles and prawns to the salad and gently mix together. Drizzle over the dressing and serve topped with extra herbs and a wedge of lime.

You can find kelp noodles in your local health food shop. They are a great addition to soups and cold salads and give you a good dose of iodine, which is a common deficiency.

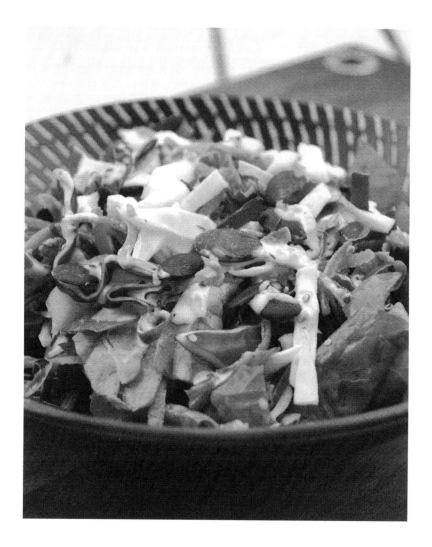

Coleslaw

SERVES 4

- 3 teaspoons Basic Mayonnaise (see recipe on above pages)

- 1 teaspoon wholegrain mustard

- juice of 1/2 lemon

- 1/4 red cabbage, shredded

- 1/4 white cabbage, shredded

- 1 medium carrot, grated

- 1 spring onion (scallion), finely chopped

- 1 handful of activated pumpkin seeds (pepitas) (see Ingredients Glossary)

- 2 handfuls of baby spinach leaves, roughly chopped

Place the Basic Mayonnaise, mustard and lemon juice in a small jar and shake until well combined.

Place all the other ingredients in a large bowl and gently toss to combine. Add the dressing just prior to serving to maintain the crispness of the coleslaw.

If we are having a busy week, this coleslaw becomes an evening staple. We make a big batch and leave it undressed (it will keep for a few days this way). It also goes really well with some hardboiled eggs—the perfect quick meal!

Cucumber Salad with Vietnamese Herbs

SERVES 2–4

- 2 tablespoons coconut oil

- 2 small Asian shallots, finely sliced (see Ingredients Glossary) or 1 medium brown onion, finely sliced

- 4 iceberg lettuce leaves, shredded

- 2 large Lebanese cucumbers, cut into thin batons

- 1 handful of mung bean shoots

- 1 handful of coriander (cilantro), roughly chopped

- 4 sawtooth coriander leaves, roughly chopped (see Ingredients Glossary)

- 1 handful of mint leaves, roughly chopped

- drizzle of Vietnamese Salad Dressing, to serve (see recipe on above pages)

Heat the coconut oil in a small saucepan over a high heat. Shallow fry the shallots until golden brown, then drain on paper towel and set aside.

In a large bowl, combine the lettuce, cucumber, mung bean shoots, coriander, sawtooth and mint. Pour a little of the Vietnamese Salad Dressing over the salad, sprinkle with fried shallots and serve.

I am obsessed with Vietnamese food. It is just so fresh, packed with flavour and simple to make.

Note: If you cannot find any sawtooth coriander, use common coriander (cilantro) leaves instead.

Lola's Fresh Sardine Salad

SERVES 4

- 1 small Lebanese cucumber, diced
- 1 punnet cherry tomatoes, halved
- 3 spring onions (scallions), finely chopped
- 1 carrot, grated
- 1 medium beetroot, scrubbed, peeled and grated
- 1/4 cup flaked almonds, toasted
- 3 tablespoons extra virgin olive oil
- zest and juice of 1 lemon
- 1 tablespoon maple syrup
- 1 clove garlic, crushed
- sea salt, to taste
- freshly ground black pepper, to taste
- 12 whole sardines, scaled and gutted
- extra virgin coconut oil, for brushing the fish
- 4 tablespoons roughly chopped flat-leaf (Italian) parsley
- 1 lemon, quartered

Place the cucumber, tomato, spring onion, carrot, beetroot and almonds in a large bowl and gently toss to combine.

In a separate small bowl, whisk together the olive oil, lemon zest and juice, maple syrup and garlic. Pour the dressing over the salad and season with salt and pepper. Mix well, then set aside until ready to serve.

Wash and pat dry the sardines. Brush with the coconut oil and season with salt and pepper all over. Heat a griddle pan, frying pan or barbecue grill and cook the sardines over a very high heat for 3–4 minutes in total, turning once. The sardines should be cooked through and slightly charred.

Divide the salad between four serving plates and top each one with three sardines. Sprinkle with parsley and squeeze over the juice from a lemon wedge.

This recipe is from Lola Berry, a fellow nutritionist and foodie. Sardines are packed with nutrients and omega-3s. If you have had a busy day and run out of time, this dish can always be made with sustainably sourced tinned sardines. This is a super healthy, quick meal.

Grilled Peach, Walnut and Beetroot Salad

SERVES 2–4

- 6–8 baby beetroot, scrubbed and quartered

- 2 peaches, halved and seeded

- 1/2 cup activated walnuts, roughly chopped (see Ingredients Glossary)

- 1 tablespoon raw honey (see Ingredients Glossary)

- 2 large handfuls of mixed salad or baby spinach leaves, roughly chopped

- 1 handful snow pea (mangetout) sprouts, chopped in 3cm (1 1/4in) lengths

- 1 small handful of activated pumpkin seeds (pepitas) (see Ingredients Glossary)

- 1 small handful of goat's feta (omit if you are sensitive to dairy or on the 28-day Reset)

- drizzle of Blueberry Balsamic Reduction, to serve (see recipe on above pages)

Preheat the oven to 200°C (400°F).

Place the beetroot quarters on a baking tray lined with baking paper and roast for 45 minutes.

While the beetroot is roasting, grill the peaches flesh-side down on a grill pan over a low to medium heat for 2–4 minutes on each side. After grilling, chop each peach half into quarters and set aside.

Once the beetroot quarters are out of the oven, set them aside to cool, leaving the oven on. Place the walnuts on the same tray the beetroots were on, with a clean sheet of baking paper. Drizzle honey over the walnuts and roast for 8 minutes.

Place the salad mix, snow pea sprouts, pumpkin seeds, beetroot and peaches in a bowl, and gently toss. Transfer the salad to a serving plate or bowl, then top with small pinches of goat's feta and the honeyed walnuts. Just prior to serving, drizzle over the Blueberry Balsamic Reduction.

This salad is so bright and colourful you can just *see* that it is full of nutrients!

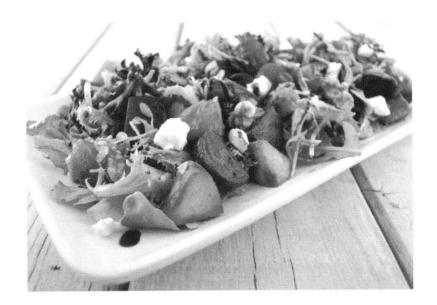

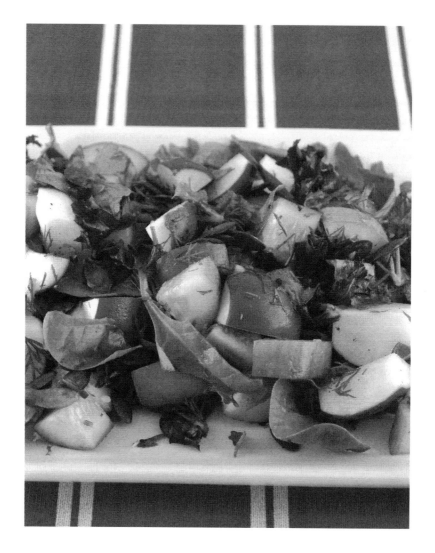

Radish Salad

SERVES 2–4

- juice of 1/2 lemon
- 1/2 teaspoon raw honey (see Ingredients Glossary)
- 2–3 tablespoons olive oil
- pinch of freshly ground black pepper

- 1 bunch of small radishes, ends trimmed and quartered

- 2 small Lebanese cucumbers, quartered lengthways and roughly chopped into 1cm (1/2in) pieces

- 2 handfuls of baby spinach leaves or mixed lettuce, roughly chopped

- 1 small handful of dill, finely chopped

- 1 small handful of activated pumpkin seeds (pepitas) (see Ingredients Glossary)

Place the lemon juice, honey, olive oil and pepper in a jar and shake well to combine.

In a bowl, combine the radish, cucumber and spinach, sprinkle in the dill and mix. Drizzle over the dressing to coat, then sprinkle with the pumpkin seeds and serve.

I love the spiciness that radish adds to a salad. If you look for nice small ones, they won't be superhot. Radishes also contain a good dose of vitamin C!

Rainbow Salad

SERVES 2–4

- 1/2 small red cabbage, shredded

- 1 red capsicum (pepper), thinly sliced

- 2 spring onions (scallions), thinly sliced
- 1 handful of snow pea (mangetout) sprouts, cut into 3cm (1 1/4in) lengths
- 2 handfuls of baby spinach leaves, roughly chopped
- 2 medium carrots, cut into thin strips
- 2 small Lebanese cucumbers, cut into thin strips
- 1/4 cup activated almonds, roughly chopped, to garnish (see Ingredients Glossary)
- drizzle of Curry Salad Dressing, to serve (see recipe on above pages)

Place all the vegetables in a large bowl and gently toss until combined.

Sprinkle over the almonds, drizzle with the Curry Salad Dressing and serve.

As the name suggests, this salad has a rainbow of colours in it! Eating a rainbow of colours ensures you get a broad range of nutrients—plus it tastes amazing.

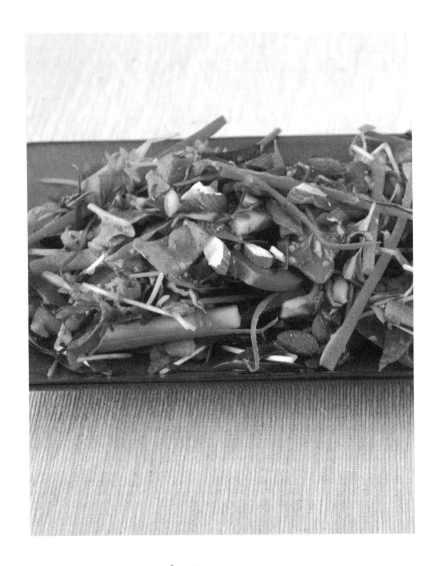

Bacon-wrapped Asparagus

SERVES 2

- 6 bacon rashers, cut into 1cm (1/2in) wide strips

- 6 asparagus spears, lower ends trimmed

- Sweet Chilli Sauce, to serve (see recipe on above pages)

306

Twist the bacon around the asparagus spears, securing with toothpicks. Grill the asparagus and bacon until cooked (about 2 or 3 minutes). Serve with the Sweet Chilli Sauce.

> The sweet chilli sauce is the secret weapon in this recipe. It works so well with the asparagus and bacon.

Sweet Potato Mash

SERVES 4

- 4 small sweet potatoes (kumara), peeled and roughly chopped
- 2 tablespoons butter or ghee (see Ingredients Glossary), at room temperature
- pink Himalayan salt, to taste (see Ingredients Glossary)
- freshly ground black pepper, to taste

Place the sweet potato in a large pot and cover with water. Bring to the boil and simmer for 10–15 minutes or until tender. Drain and transfer to a bowl. Add the butter and mash until smooth. Season with salt and pepper and serve.

> Great in winter, there is something so decadent about a good mash with lashings of butter. And you

get to eat this one guilt free, because butter is good for you!

Sweet Potato Fritters

MAKES 8–12

- 1 medium sweet potato (kumara), peeled and grated
- 1 large zucchini (courgette), grated
- 1 spring onion (scallion), finely chopped
- 1 long red chilli, seeded and finely chopped
- 1 large handful of baby spinach leaves, roughly chopped
- 1/2 teaspoon ground nutmeg
- 1/2 teaspoon ground cinnamon
- freshly ground black pepper, to taste
- 4 eggs
- butter or ghee (see Ingredients Glossary), for frying

Combine the sweet potato and zucchini in a large bowl, squeezing out any excess water with your hands. Add the remaining ingredients, except the butter, and mix until well combined.

Melt a small amount of butter in a frying pan over a low to medium heat. Place large tablespoons of the mixture into the pan and cook each side for about 5 minutes or until golden brown. Cook four to five at a time and repeat with the remaining mixture.

Serve hot or cold as part of a meal or with salad.

> These guys make great lunchbox treats. They are equally tasty cold or hot and you can leave out the chilli if you want to give them to the kids.

Tip: These fritters go very well with my Avocado Salsa (see recipe on above pages).

Sweet Potato Salad

SERVES 4–6

- 1 large sweet potato (kumara), peeled and cubed
- 1/4 teaspoon ground nutmeg
- 1/2 teaspoon ground cumin
- freshly ground black pepper, to taste
- 1 tablespoon coconut oil
- 1 tablespoon raw honey (see Ingredients Glossary)
- 2–3 handfuls of mixed salad leaves or baby spinach leaves, roughly chopped

- 1 handful of snow pea (mangetout) sprouts, chopped into 3cm (1 1/4in) lengths

- 6 baby zucchini (courgettes), peeled to make thin slivers

- 6 asparagus spears, lower ends trimmed and discarded and the rest peeled to make thin slivers

- drizzle of Honey Wholegrain Mustard Dressing, to serve (see recipe on above pages)

- 1 handful of activated pumpkin seeds (pepitas) (see Ingredients Glossary)

Preheat the oven to 180°C (350°F).

Line a roasting tray with baking paper.

Place the sweet potato in a large bowl and sprinkle with the ground nutmeg, ground cumin and pepper and mix well.

In a small bowl combine the coconut oil and honey, then pour the mix over the sweet potato and stir through, making sure all of the sweet potato is coated. Spread the sweet potato evenly over the tray and cook for 20 minutes or until golden brown, turning once during baking. Remove from the oven and set aside to cool.

Place the mixed lettuce leaves, snow pea sprouts, zucchini and asparagus in a bowl and gently hand toss.

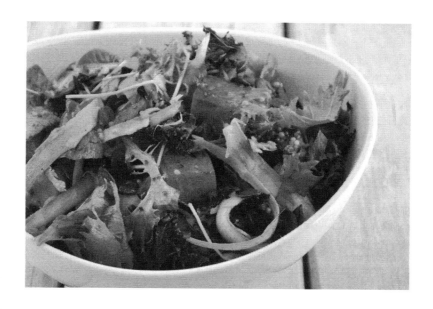

Add the sweet potato to the salad, drizzle with the Honey Wholegrain Mustard Dressing and gently mix. Sprinkle with the pumpkin seeds and serve.

This salad is a crowd pleaser at any BBQ I take it to—sneaky Paleo! Use a potato peeler to peel the zucchini and asparagus into thin slivers.

Roasted Eggplant, Cauliflower and Warm Chicken Salad

SERVES 4

- 1 large eggplant (aubergine), cubed

- 1 tablespoon coconut oil or ghee (see Ingredients Glossary)

- large pinch of pink Himalayan salt (see Ingredients Glossary)

- large pinch of freshly ground black pepper

- pinch of chilli flakes

- 3 cloves garlic, crushed

- 1 punnet grape tomatoes, halved

- 1 tablespoon butter or ghee (see Ingredients Glossary)

- 2 chicken breasts, cut into chunks

- 1/2 medium brown onion, finely chopped

- 1/2 large head of cauliflower, grated

- 1 small handful of flat-leaf (Italian) parsley, finely chopped

- 1 small handful of basil, finely chopped

- 1 tablespoon olive oil

- juice of 1 lemon

- 1 small handful of baby spinach leaves, roughly chopped

- 1 small handful goat's feta, crumbled, to serve (omit if you are sensitive to dairy or on the 28-day Reset)

Preheat the oven to 200°C (400°F). Line two baking trays with baking paper.

Place the eggplant in a bowl, mix through the coconut oil, then add the salt, pepper, chilli flakes and garlic. Mix well, then turn out onto a baking tray and roast for 20–30 minutes, turning once.

As the eggplant is cooking, place the tomatoes on the second tray and roast for 15 minutes.

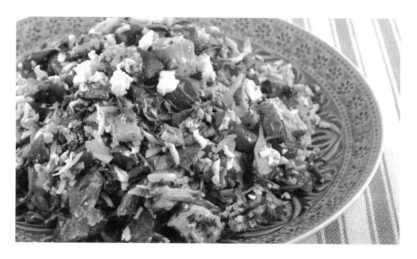

Melt the butter in a pan over a medium heat and brown the chicken until cooked through. Turn out onto a plate to cool.

In the same pan brown the onion until soft, then add the cauliflower and stir for a few minutes. Take off the heat and allow to cool in the pan for 5 minutes. Add the parsley and basil to the cauliflower and mix together.

Place the olive oil and lemon juice in a small jar and shake until well combined.

Gently toss the roasted eggplant, roasted tomato, chicken, cauliflower mix and spinach in a large bowl until combined. Drizzle with the lemon and olive oil and serve with the goat's feta sprinkled on top.

> All I can say is yum, yum, yum! This is a wonderful, tasty warm salad.

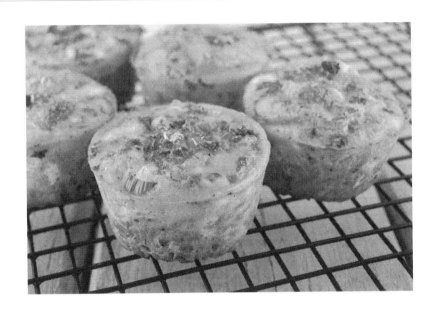

Egg and Mince Muffins

SERVES 2–3

- butter or ghee (see Ingredients Glossary), for greasing
- 1 1/2 cups Asian Mince (see recipe on below pages)
- 6 eggs, whisked
- pink Himalayan salt, to taste (see Ingredients Glossary)

- freshly ground black pepper, to taste

- 1 handful of broccoli florets, cut into small pieces

- 1 asparagus spear, lower end trimmed and discarded and the rest cut into 2mm (1/16in) disks

- 1 small handful of flat-leaf (Italian) parsley, finely chopped

- 1–2 tablespoons nutritional yeast (see Ingredients Glossary)

Preheat the oven to 180°C (350°F).

Rub the butter into six cups of a large muffin tray. Divide the mince evenly into the bottom of each muffin cup, then pour a small amount of the egg mix on top. Gently mix with a fork to ensure the egg gets between the mince so the muffin stays together. Season with salt and pepper.

Place the broccoli and asparagus onto the mix, then divide the remaining egg mixture evenly over the top of the muffins and sprinkle each with some parsley and nutritional yeast.

Bake for 25–30 minutes or until the egg has set. Serve hot or cold.

> This is another one of my husband's favourites. He'll happily eat these for breakfast, lunch and dinner.

Oysters with Salsa and Red Wine Vinaigrette

SERVES 2–4

- 12 small grape tomatoes, diced
- 1/2 red (Spanish) onion, diced
- 1 small bunch of flat-leaf (Italian) parsley, finely chopped
- 12 oysters, shucked
- drizzle of Red Wine Vinaigrette (see recipe on above pages)

Mix the tomato and onion in a bowl until well combined. Stir through the parsley, then enough vinaigrette to coat the tomatoes well. Place a small amount of the tomato and onion mix on top of each oyster and serve.

When choosing oysters, nothing beats fresh. As with all seafood, they should smell like salty sea air. Oysters are an excellent source of selenium and zinc, which are common deficiencies.

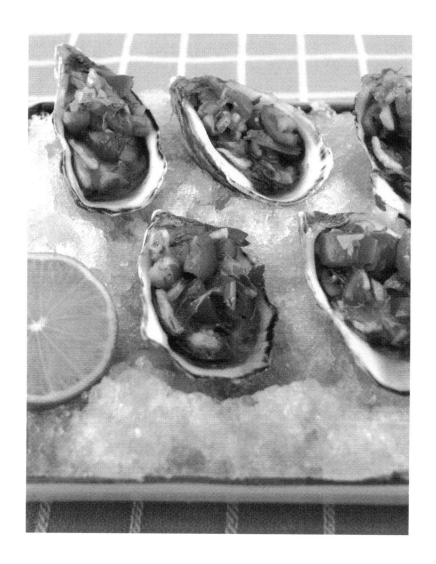

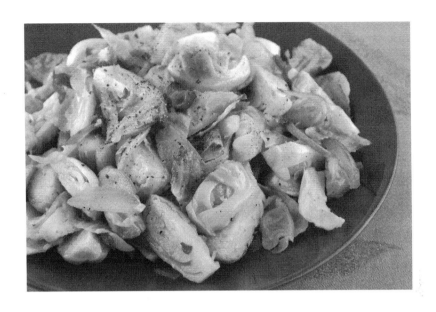

Best-ever Brussels

SERVES 2

- 2–3 tablespoons butter

- 1 clove garlic, finely chopped

- 1/2 red (Spanish) onion, finely sliced

- 1/4 long red chilli, seeded and finely chopped

- 12–14 brussels sprouts, ends trimmed and quartered

- pink Himalayan salt, to taste (see Ingredients Glossary)

- freshly ground black pepper, to taste

Melt 1 tablespoon of the butter in a pan over a medium heat. Add the garlic and onion and sauté until soft. Add the chilli and sauté until fragrant then add the rest of the butter and the brussels sprouts and cook for a further 6 minutes or until the brussels sprouts are tender. Serve seasoned with salt and black pepper.

If you think you hate brussels sprouts, you have not tried this recipe! Guaranteed to make you fall in love with eating brussels sprouts!

Broccoli and Chicken Salad

SERVES 2

- 1 tablespoon butter or ghee (see Ingredients Glossary)
- 1 chicken breast
- freshly ground black pepper, to taste
- 1 head of broccoli, chopped into small florets and stem diced
- 2 handfuls of baby spinach leaves, roughly chopped
- 1 handful of snow peas (mangetout), ends trimmed and halved
- 1 handful of activated macadamia nuts, roughly chopped (see Ingredients Glossary)

- drizzle of Honey Wholegrain Mustard Dressing, to serve (see recipe on above pages)

Melt the butter in a pan over a medium heat.

Season the chicken breast with pepper, then fry in the pan until brown on both sides and cooked through. Set aside to cool.

While the chicken is cooling, mix the broccoli, spinach, snow peas and macadamia nuts in a bowl. Slice the chicken and mix through the salad. Drizzle with the Honey Wholegrain Mustard Dressing and serve.

There are vegetables that people always eat cooked or steamed and they are equally yummy, if not more so, eaten raw! Broccoli is fantastic in salads—and don't throw away the stems, they are so juicy and sweet!

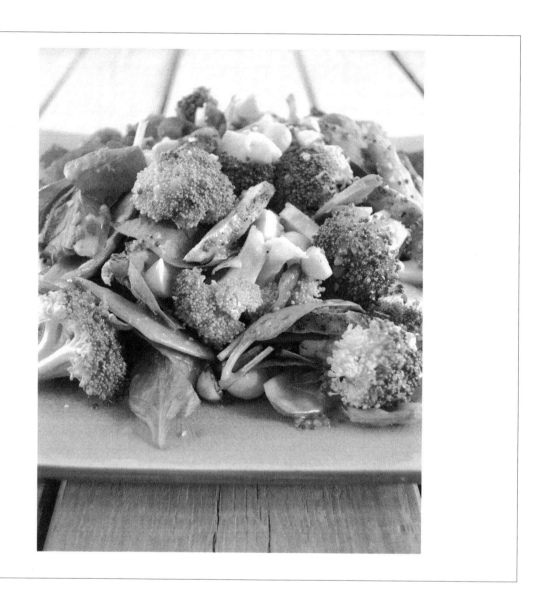

Larger meals

Asian Mince Breakfast Omelette

SERVES 2

- 1 tablespoon butter

- 4 bacon rashers, roughly chopped

- 300g (10 1/2oz) Asian Mince (see recipe on below pages)

- 6 eggs

- freshly ground black pepper, to taste

- 1/2 teaspoon coconut aminos or tamari sauce (see Ingredients Glossary for both)

- 1 large handful of baby spinach leaves, roughly chopped

Melt the butter in a pan over a medium heat. Add the bacon and fry on both sides until cooked then add the cold (leftover) mince.

While the mince is warming through, add the eggs to a bowl and whisk with a fork. Add the pepper and coconut aminos to the eggs, then the spinach and mix through. Pour the egg mix evenly over the mince and cook for 5 minutes or until the egg is cooked through. Serve immediately.

Many of the meals I make for breakfast are quite large! This is because it sets you up right for the rest of the day—try it and see how you feel.

Bun-free Burgers

MAKES 4 BURGERS

Burger Patties

- butter or ghee (see Ingredients Glossary), for frying

- 1/2 brown onion, finely chopped

- 2 cloves garlic, finely chopped

- 1 egg

- 1 small handful of flat-leaf (Italian) parsley, finely chopped

- 500g (1lb 2oz) beef mince

- 2 bacon rashers

- 1 teaspoon tomato paste

- 1/4 teaspoon pink Himalayan salt (see Ingredients Glossary)

- 1 teaspoon freshly ground black pepper

- 1 tablespoon Dijon mustard

- 1/2 teaspoon chilli powder

- 1/2 zucchini (courgette), sliced lengthways

- 1 small eggplant (aubergine), sliced into rounds

- coconut oil, for brushing

- 4 iceberg lettuce leaves, well washed, to serve

- Dijon Mustard Mayonnaise, to serve (see recipe on above pages)

- Lacto-fermented Sauerkraut, to serve (see recipe on above pages)

Melt the butter in a frying pan over a medium heat. Add the onion and garlic and cook until brown, then set aside to cool.

In a food processor, combine all the other patty ingredients with the cooled onion and garlic and pulse until well combined. Using your hands, divide the mixture into four equal portions and mould into balls.

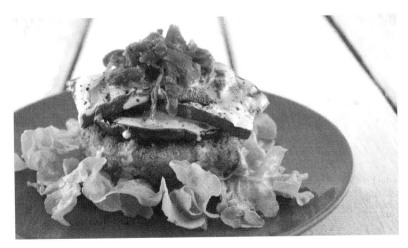

In the same frying pan, melt some more butter over a medium heat. Place the meat in the pan, flatten with a spatula to make flat patties, and cook on both sides for 5 minutes or until golden brown and cooked through. Rest them on a chopping board covered with foil once cooked.

While the patties are cooking, brush the zucchini and eggplant with coconut oil and season with pepper. On a grill pan over a medium to high heat, grill the vegetables on both sides then set aside.

To build the burgers, place each patty on a lettuce leaf, adding slices of eggplant and zucchini and top with Dijon mustard mayonnaise and sauerkraut.

My inspiration for these bun-free burgers actually came from a bratwurst hotdog my husband had when we were on holiday. The Dijon mustard mayonnaise and sauerkraut work really well with the burger!

Asian Mince in Lettuce Cups

SERVES 6

Asian Mince
- 2 carrots, grated
- 1 zucchini (courgette), grated
- 1 tablespoon butter
- 1 brown onion, finely chopped

- 2–3 cloves garlic, finely chopped (depending on how strong you like the garlic)

- 1 large red chilli, seeded and chopped

- 500g (1lb 2oz) beef mince

- 500g (1lb 2oz) pork mince

- 2 tablespoons coconut aminos or tamari sauce (see Ingredients Glossary for both)

- 2 tablespoons fish sauce

- 3 tablespoons tomato paste

- freshly ground black pepper, to taste

- 1 spring onion (scallion), finely chopped

- 1 handful of coriander (cilantro), roughly chopped

- 1 quantity of Asian Egg Crêpes (see recipe on above pages), cut into strips

- 4–6 iceberg lettuce leaves, to serve

Place the carrot and zucchini in a bowl and, using your hands, squeeze out any excess liquid.

Melt the butter in a frying pan over a medium heat, add the onion and garlic and sauté until soft. Add the chilli and fry for 5 minutes or until the flavours come out, then add the mince and cook for a further 5 minutes.

Add the carrot, zucchini, coconut aminos, fish sauce, tomato paste and pepper and cook until most of the liquid is gone (about 10 minutes).

Take the pan off the heat and stir through the spring onion, coriander and egg crêpe strips.

Serve using the lettuce leaves as cups for the mince.

Tip: Any leftovers can be used the following day to make the Asian Mince Breakfast Omelette (see recipe on above pages) for breakfast or the Egg and Mince Muffins (see recipe on above pages).

This recipe has to be one of my favourites. It is quick to make, full of flavour and the leftovers are so versatile!

Cauliflower and Sweet Potato Soup

SERVES 6

- butter or ghee (see Ingredients Glossary), for frying
- 2 leeks, white part only, roughly chopped
- 2 cloves garlic, roughly chopped
- 1 small sweet potato (kumara), peeled and roughly chopped
- 1 head of cauliflower, roughly chopped
- 800ml (28fl oz) chicken stock

- 400ml (14fl oz) full-fat coconut milk

- 1 tablespoon horseradish cream or 1 teaspoon fresh horseradish, grated (see Ingredients Glossary)

- freshly ground black pepper, to taste

- 2 tablespoons chives, finely chopped, to garnish

- 1 slice smoked salmon, cut into slivers, to garnish

- 1 teaspoon truffle oil, to garnish (see Ingredients Glossary)

Melt a knob of butter in a large heavy-based pot over a medium heat. Add the leek and garlic and cook until the leek is soft but not brown. Add the sweet potato, cauliflower, chicken stock and coconut milk, bring to the boil then reduce the heat and simmer, covered, for 25 minutes or until the cauliflower and sweet potato are soft. Take the pot off the heat and blend the soup until smooth using a hand blender. Stir through the horseradish cream and season with pepper.

Serve in bowls, topped with chives, a sliver of salmon and a small drizzle of truffle oil.

A simple yet tasty soup. The cauliflower makes it velvety, rich and creamy, without the assistance of dairy cream. If you have not tried truffle oil—get some! I joke that truffle oil is Nature's MSG. It makes everything taste that little bit special.

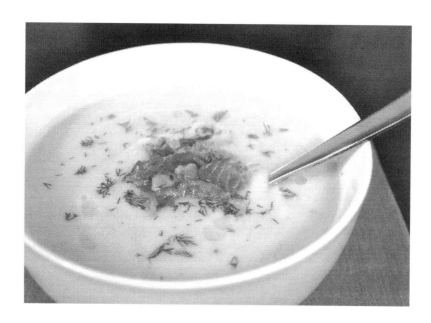

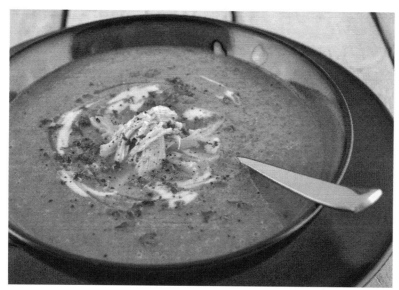

Spinach and Leek Soup

SERVES 6

- 2 tablespoons butter or ghee (see Ingredients Glossary)

- 2 leeks, white parts only, roughly chopped

- 3–4 cloves garlic, roughly chopped

- 4 sticks celery, roughly chopped

- 1/2 small head of cauliflower, roughly chopped

- 2 medium heads of broccoli, stem included, roughly chopped

- 8 cups vegetable stock

- 2 large handfuls of baby spinach leaves, roughly chopped

- 1 large handful of flat-leaf (Italian) parsley, roughly chopped, plus extra to garnish

- pinch of ground nutmeg

- freshly ground black pepper, to taste

- 1 tablespoon coconut cream (or dairy cream), to garnish

- drizzle of truffle oil, to garnish (see Ingredients Glossary)

Heat the butter in a pot over a medium heat. Add the leek and garlic and cook until the leek is soft but not brown. Add the celery, cauliflower and broccoli and cook for a further 5 minutes. Add the vegetable stock and bring to the boil, then turn down the heat and simmer for 10–15 minutes or until the cauliflower and broccoli are soft. Add the spinach and parsley and take off the heat (you want them to retain their bright green colour). Blend the mixture to a smooth consistency using a hand blender. Add nutmeg and pepper to taste.

Serve in bowls with a dollop of coconut cream, a sprinkle of parsley and a small drizzle of truffle oil.

> A beautiful, rich green soup, packed with good stuff. The flavours develop more over a few days. It also freezes well so is a great standby for a quick and easy meal.

Tip: Turn this soup into a quick complete meal by grabbing a hot chicken on the way home and adding the flaked breast to the soup, as pictured.

Nori Rolls

MAKES 6

Steamed Chicken Breast
- 1 tablespoon coconut aminos or tamari sauce, plus 2 tablespoons extra, to serve (see Ingredients Glossary for both)

- 1 tablespoon fish sauce

- juice of 1 small lime

- 1 teaspoon apple cider vinegar

- 1/2 long red chilli, seeded and finely chopped, plus extra to serve

- 3–4 kaffir lime leaves, finely chopped

- 1/2 teaspoon raw honey (see Ingredients Glossary)

- 2 chicken breasts

- 1 quantity of Asian Egg Crêpes (see recipe on above pages), cut into strips

- 1–2 cucumbers, julienned

- 1 carrot, julienned

- 1 small red capsicum (pepper), finely sliced

- 1 spring onion (scallion), finely chopped

- 6 nori sheets (see Ingredients Glossary)

- 1 bamboo rolling mat

- 3 tablespoons Horseradish Mayonnaise (see recipe on above pages)

- Sweet Chilli Sauce, to serve (see recipe on above pages)

In a small bowl, combine the coconut aminos, fish sauce, lime juice, apple cider vinegar, chilli, kaffir lime leaves and honey.

Place the chicken breasts on two separate pieces of baking paper, pour the combined sauce over the chicken, then fold each side of the baking paper over the chicken to form a parcel. Place the sealed parcels in a bamboo steamer over a pot of boiling water and steam for 15 minutes or until cooked through. Once the chicken is cooked, allow to cool and then finely slice.

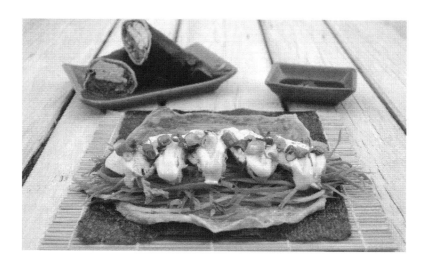

Place the egg crêpe strips, cucumber, carrot, capsicum and spring onion on separate plates to assemble the rolls. To assemble the rolls, place a nori sheet on the bamboo rolling mat and add some egg crêpe, cucumber, carrot, capsicum and chicken along the middle of the sheet. Add a dollop of Horseradish Mayonnaise and some spring onion, then roll up the nori sheet using the bamboo rolling mat. Moisten the closing end of the nori sheet with water to stick.

Cut the roll in half and serve with the extra coconut aminos and the Sweet Chilli Sauce.

These nori rolls are so tasty you will never want to buy store-bought ones again!

Salmon and Cauli Fried Rice

SERVES 4

- 1 tablespoon ghee (see Ingredients Glossary)
- 1 medium brown onion, finely chopped
- 2 cloves garlic, minced
- 1/2 head of cauliflower, grated
- 1 red capsicum (pepper), finely sliced lengthways
- 1 handful of snow peas (mangetout), ends trimmed and roughly chopped
- 1 teaspoon coconut aminos or tamari sauce (see Ingredients Glossary for both)
- 2 spring onions (scallions), finely chopped
- 1 handful of coriander (cilantro), plus extra to serve
- freshly ground black pepper, to taste
- 4 salmon fillets, skin on
- Sweet Chilli Sauce, to serve (see recipe on above pages)

Heat the ghee in a frying pan over a medium heat. Fry the onion and garlic until the onion is soft, then add the cauliflower and stir-fry for 2 minutes. Add the capsicum, snow peas and stir-fry for a further 2 minutes, then pour over the coconut aminos and stir through. Stir in the spring onion and coriander, add the pepper and set aside.

Season the salmon fillets with black pepper and cook the fish skin-side down in the pan over a medium to high heat for 3–4 minutes until crisp. Turn and cook the other side for a further 2–3 minutes until the fish is still slightly rare in the centre.

Serve the salmon on a bed of cauli rice, topped with a few coriander leaves and Sweet Chilli Sauce.

> This is a fresh and fragrant dish that will win over even the most sceptical diners. It is also a great way to up your omega-3 intake!

Mackerel Plaki

SERVES 2

- 4 tablespoons extra virgin olive oil
- 2 small brown onions, finely chopped
- 1 large red capsicum (pepper), finely chopped
- sea salt or Celtic salt, to taste
- 3 cloves garlic, finely chopped
- 2 tablespoons flat-leaf (Italian) parsley, roughly chopped
- 2 whole mackerels, cleaned and gutted

- 1 punnet cherry tomatoes, cut in half

- 3 bay leaves

- 2 medium carrots, thinly sliced

- juice and zest of 1 lemon, plus extra zest

- 1/2 teaspoon freshly ground black pepper

- 1 cup dry white wine

Preheat the oven to 180°C (350°F).

Line a deep baking tray with foil, making sure the sides are well covered.

Place the olive oil in a frying pan and cook the onion and capsicum over a low to medium heat until softened and slightly caramelised. Season with the salt.

Stuff some of the garlic and parsley inside the fish and set aside.

Spoon half of the cooked onion and capsicum mixture on the tray and top with half the tomato, a little more garlic, bay leaves, half the carrots and half the lemon zest and lemon juice. Sprinkle with the pepper and extra salt.

Place the fish on top of the vegetables and cover with the rest of the tomato, garlic and carrots. Drizzle over the remaining lemon juice and lemon zest and pour over the wine. Cover with another piece of foil and bake, covered, for 20 minutes, letting the fish steam inside and 20 minutes, uncovered, to get some caramelisation and browning. Serve immediately.

This mackerel recipe is from the lovely Irey Macri of Eat Drink Paleo. Have a look at her website and cookbook for more amazing Paleo recipes. This recipe is based on a traditional Greek-style baked fish dish. You can add olives, sliced fennel and other herbs such as oregano or basil to the fish, if you like.

Omelette

SERVES 2–4

- butter, for frying

- 1/2 brown onion, finely chopped

- 1 clove garlic, minced

- 1/2 long red chilli, seeded and finely chopped

- 2 bacon rashers, roughly chopped

- 1/2 zucchini (courgette), diced

- 6 asparagus spears, ends trimmed and discarded, and the rest chopped into 1cm (1/2in) lengths (reserve the tips)

- 1 handful of grape tomatoes, halved

- 8 eggs

- splash of almond milk (see recipe on above pages)

- 1 large handful of baby spinach leaves, roughly chopped

- 1 handful of flat-leaf (Italian) parsley, finely chopped

- pink Himalayan salt, to taste (see Ingredients Glossary)

- freshly ground black pepper, to taste

- 4 pinches of goat's feta (omit if you are sensitive to dairy or on 28-day Reset)

- 1 spring onion (scallion), finely chopped

Melt the butter in a pan over a medium heat. Add the onion, garlic and chilli and sauté until the onion softens. Add the bacon and cook for about 5 minutes, then add the zucchini and asparagus and cook for a further 5 minutes or until the zucchini starts to soften slightly. Add the tomatoes and stir.

Crack the eggs into a bowl, add the almond milk and whisk with a fork. Add the spinach and parsley to the eggs, season with salt and pepper and mix through. Pour the egg mixture into the pan over the vegetables and bacon mix, add the reserved asparagus tips, sprinkle the goat's feta and spring onion on top and cook on a low to medium heat for about 15 minutes or until cooked through. Serve immediately.

338

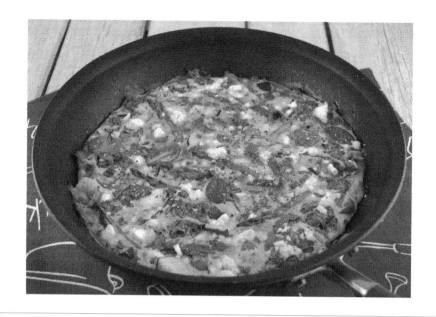

This omelette makes a regular appearance on our breakfast table. As I have mentioned before, we love to have a BIG breakfast, so this serves just the two of us!

Tip: To get a nice finish, place the pan under the grill for a few minutes until the top is golden brown.

Paleo Pizza

SERVES 2–4

- butter, for frying
- 1 1/2 bacon rashers, roughly chopped
- 1 cup butternut pumpkin, cut into 1cm (1/2in) cubes
- 2–3 tablespoons tomato paste

- 1 Paleo Pizza Base (see recipe on above pages)

- 1 small red (Spanish) onion, finely chopped

- 10 small slices of free-range salami

- 1/2 red capsicum (pepper), finely chopped

- 1/2 yellow capsicum (pepper), finely chopped

- 1/4 zucchini (courgette), finely chopped

- 5 pieces marinated artichoke (seed oil free), roughly chopped (see Ingredients Glossary)

- 1 long red chilli, seeded and finely chopped

- 6–7 pinches of goat's feta (omit if you are sensitive to dairy or on 28-day Reset)

- 2–3 teaspoons of Basil Pesto (see recipe on above pages)

Preheat the oven to 180°C (350°F).

Place a little butter in a frying pan and cook the bacon as desired.

Steam the pumpkin until tender and set aside.

Spread the tomato paste evenly over the pizza base, then add all the other toppings, except the goat's feta and Basil Pesto. Evenly place small pinches of feta and dollops of basil pesto over the pizza, then bake for 15–20 minutes.

340

This is one of our favourite pizza combinations. The trick is to make sure the base is loaded with vegetables. Get the kids to help with the toppings—they are far more likely to eat something if they have been involved in the cooking process.

Tip: This is just one of hundreds of different pizzas you can make. Don't be afraid to try other combinations of your favourite vegetables and meats.

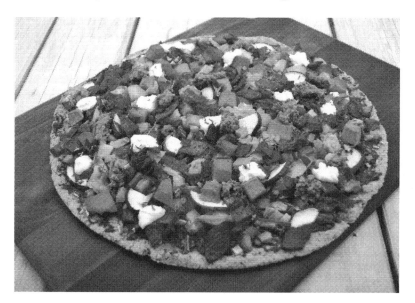

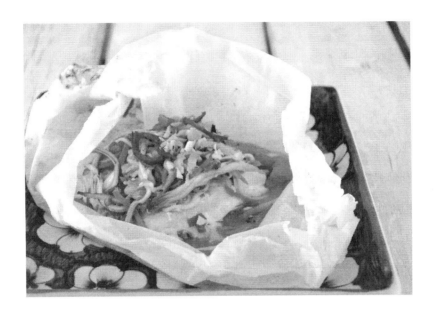

Asian Fish En Papillote

SERVES 4

- 4 white fish fillets

- 2 large zucchini (courgettes), julienned

- 2 large carrots, julienned

- 2 spring onions (scallions), finely chopped

- 2cm (3/4in) piece of fresh ginger, peeled and cut into batons

- juice of 1 lime

- 2 cloves garlic, finely sliced

- 2 tablespoons fish sauce

- 1 teaspoon sesame oil

- 1/2 long red chilli, seeded and finely sliced
- freshly ground black pepper, to taste

Preheat the oven to 200°C (400°F).

Set out four pieces of baking paper on a flat surface and place a piece of fish in the middle of each one.

In a bowl, combine the zucchini, carrot and spring onion and place equal quantities of the mixed vegetables on top of each piece of fish.

In a small bowl, combine the ginger, lime juice, garlic, fish sauce, sesame oil, chilli and pepper, and evenly divide the mixture over each fish parcel.

Close the parcels by folding over the baking paper, making sure the edges are sealed, and bake for 10–15 minutes or until the fish is cooked through.

Serve on a bed of steamed vegetables, such as bok choy or cauliflower and broccoli florets.

> In French, *en papillote* simply means 'in parchment'. It is a method of cooking where food is put in a parcel and baked. It works really well with the fish and allows all of the flavours to develop nicely while cooking.

Avocado Salsa and Salmon

SERVES 2

- 2 salmon steaks

- coconut oil, for brushing

- freshly ground black pepper, to taste

- 1 quantity of Avocado Salsa (see recipe on above pages)

- pinch of finely chopped flat-leaf (Italian) parsley, to garnish

Heat a grill pan over a medium heat. Rub the salmon with some coconut oil and season on both sides with pepper. Cook the salmon for 2 minutes on each side or until a little pink inside.

Serve the Avocado Salsa with salmon flaked over the top. Garnish with the parsley and extra black pepper.

This meal really packs a punch in the good fats department, combined with loads of anti-inflammatory goodness!

Tip: This meal is yummy served cold, and you can make double for the next day's lunch.

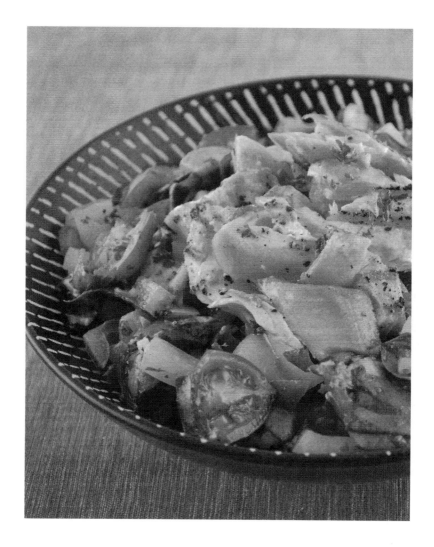

Prawn Laksa

SERVES 4–6

Laksa Paste

- 1 tablespoon coriander seeds

- 1 tablespoon cumin seeds

- 2 lemongrass sticks, white part only

- 4–6 long red chillies, seeded and finely chopped
- 1 teaspoon ground turmeric
- 3cm (1 1/4in) piece of fresh ginger, roughly chopped
- 3 cloves garlic, roughly chopped
- 3 Asian shallots (see Ingredients Glossary) or 1 brown onion, roughly chopped
- 8 activated macadamia nuts, roughly chopped (see Ingredients Glossary)
- 1 tablespoon shrimp paste
- 1 tablespoon lime juice
- 2 tablespoons coconut oil
- 700ml (24fl oz) chicken stock
- 400ml (14fl oz) coconut milk
- 4 kaffir lime leaves
- 2 tablespoons fish sauce
- 1 tablespoon coconut sugar (see Ingredients Glossary)
- juice of 1 large lime
- 1 large carrot, julienned (reserve some to garnish)
- 1 large zucchini (courgette), cut into batons
- 1 bunch of bok choy, roughly chopped

- 700g (1lb 9oz) raw medium prawns, peeled and deveined with tail intact

- 1 handful of mung bean shoots

- 1 handful of snow peas (mangetout) sprouts, ends trimmed and finely sliced

- 1 small handful of coriander (cilantro), roughly chopped, to garnish

- 2 limes, cut into wedges, to serve

First make the laksa paste. Dry-roast the coriander and cumin seeds separately in a dry frying pan over a medium heat until they become fragrant, then add them to a mortar and pestle and grind to a powder.

Lightly crush the lemongrass with the flat of a knife. In a blender or food processor, place the lemongrass, chilli, turmeric, ginger, garlic, Asian shallots, macadamia nuts, shrimp paste, lime juice and ground coriander and cumin, and blend into a paste.

Heat the coconut oil in a large pot over a low heat and cook the paste for about 5 minutes or until fragrant. Add the stock and bring to the boil, then turn down the heat and simmer for 10 minutes. Add the coconut milk, kaffir lime leaves, fish sauce, coconut sugar and lime juice and simmer for another 5 minutes. Add the carrot, zucchini and bok choy and simmer for 1 minute, then add the prawns and simmer for a further 2 minutes.

Place a small handful of mung bean shoots in the bottom of every serving bowl. Ladle the laksa into the bowls and top with the snow pea sprouts, reserved carrot and coriander leaves. Serve with lime wedges.

My husband loves a good prawn laksa and this creation passed the test with flying colours. You can make a double batch of laksa paste and store it in an airtight container in the fridge for a few months.

Dukkah-crusted Chicken Thighs

SERVES 2–3

- coconut oil, for greasing
- 1 egg
- Dukkah Mix (see recipe on above pages)
- 6 chicken thighs, halved
- Garlic Aioli Mayonnaise, to serve (see recipe on above pages)

Preheat the oven to 180°C (350°F).

Line a baking tray with baking paper and grease with the coconut oil.

Whisk the egg with a fork to make an egg wash.

Dip the chicken pieces in the egg wash, then coat them with the Dukkah Mix, making sure they are well coated (any remaining Dukkah Mix must be thrown away as it is now contaminated with raw chicken and egg).

Place on the baking tray and bake for 20–30 minutes or until the juices run clear (you can then place them under the grill for 5 minutes if you want to give the chicken a nice crunchy coating).

Serve with a salad and some Garlic Aioli Mayonnaise.

> These little chicken thigh bites are tasty hot and cold. They make great lunches the next day, tossed through a salad.

Chicken Stuffed with Basil Pesto and Semi-sundried Tomatoes

SERVES 2

- 2 chicken breasts

- 2 tablespoons Basil Pesto (see recipe on above pages)

- 6 semi-sundried tomatoes

- 2 bacon rashers

- 1 tablespoon butter or ghee (see Ingredients Glossary)

Preheat the oven to 175°C (325°F).

Line a baking tray with baking paper.

Cut a slit in the chicken breasts and stuff 1 tablespoon of the Basil Pesto and three sundried tomatoes into each one. Wrap each chicken breast with a rasher of bacon with the ends meeting under the breast.

Melt the butter in a pan over a medium heat and cook the chicken breasts, bottom side down to seal the bases for about 3 minutes. Gently turn over and brown the top.

Place the chicken breasts on the baking tray and bake for 20–30 minutes or until the juices run clear.

Serve with your favourite salad.

This dish is super quick to prepare and very tasty.

White Fish Stew

SERVES 4–6

- butter or ghee (see Ingredients Glossary), for frying
- 1 large brown onion, sliced
- 4 cloves garlic, finely chopped
- 2 large carrots, roughly chopped
- 1 large zucchini (courgette), roughly chopped

- 1 small sweet potato (kumara), peeled and roughly chopped

- 1 long red chilli, seeded and finely chopped

- 2 sticks celery, chopped

- 1 cup good red wine, optional

- 1x400g (14oz) tin whole tomatoes

- 2 tablespoons tomato paste

- 2 teaspoons dried oregano

- 1 teaspoon dried basil

- 1 teaspoon ground coriander

- 1/2 teaspoon ground cumin

- pinch of pink Himalayan salt (see Ingredients Glossary)

- freshly ground black pepper, to taste

- 4 white fish fillets, cut into bite-sized pieces

- 1 handful of flat-leaf (Italian) parsley, finely chopped

- 1 handful of coriander (cilantro), finely chopped

Melt the butter in a large heavy-based pot over a medium heat. Add the onion and garlic and sauté until soft. Add the carrot, zucchini, sweet potato, chilli and celery and sauté to infuse all the flavours and to start the cooking process.

Add the wine and simmer for 2 minutes or until some of the wine evaporates, then add the tinned tomatoes, tomato paste, oregano, basil, ground coriander, cumin, salt and pepper, stirring well. Simmer, uncovered, for about 15 minutes.

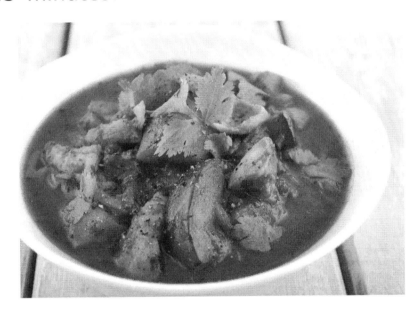

Add the fish pieces and stir through gently. Simmer, uncovered, for a further 5–7 minutes or until the fish looks opaque and is cooked through. Stir in the parsley and coriander and serve.

You can leave the wine out of this stew if you prefer. Because the fish only needs to be cooked for a moment, this stew is quick and easy to put together.

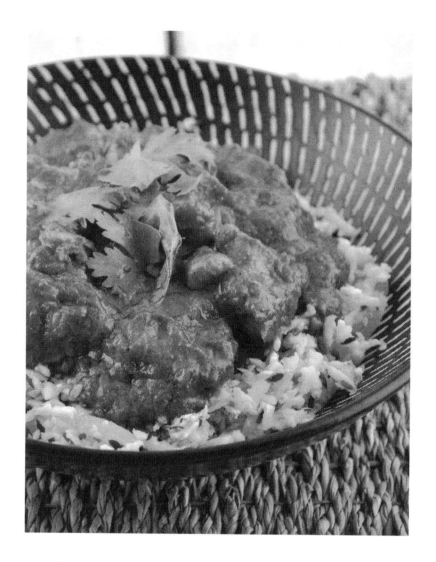

Butter Chicken

SERVES 6

- 3 tablespoons butter

- 1kg (2lb 4oz) chicken thighs, deboned and cut into chunks

- 1 tablespoon grated fresh ginger

- 1 clove garlic, finely chopped

- 2 teaspoons ground coriander

- 2 teaspoons ground cumin

- 1 teaspoon garam masala

- 1/4 teaspoon chilli powder

- 1x400g (14oz) tin whole tomatoes

- 2 tablespoons tomato paste

- 1/2 cup coconut cream

- 1 small handful of coriander (cilantro), roughly chopped, to garnish

- 1 quantity of Cumin-spiced Cauliflower Rice, to serve (see recipe on above pages)

Melt 1 tablespoon of the butter in a pan over a high heat. Add the chicken in batches and cook until brown, then set aside (do not completely cook the chicken through, just brown it).

Turn the pan down to a medium heat and add the remaining butter, ginger and garlic, and cook for 2 minutes or until fragrant. Add the ground coriander, cumin, garam masala and chilli powder, stir for 30 seconds, then add the tinned tomatoes and tomato paste and simmer for 10 minutes. Return the chicken to the pan and stir through the coconut cream. Simmer for a further 10 minutes or until the chicken is cooked through.

Sprinkle over the fresh coriander and serve on a bed of Cumin-spiced Cauliflower Rice.

As with all curries, the flavours develop overnight, so this butter chicken is divine the next day!

Chicken Meatloaf

SERVES 8

- 1 large zucchini (courgette), grated
- 1 large carrot, grated
- 1 parsnip, grated
- 500g (1lb 2oz) chicken mince
- 3 bacon rashers
- 3 eggs
- 1 large red chilli
- 1 small brown onion, roughly chopped
- 3 cloves garlic, roughly chopped
- pink Himalayan salt, to taste (see Ingredients Glossary)
- freshly ground black pepper, to taste
- 1 small handful of flat-leaf (Italian) parsley
- 1 spring onion (scallion), roughly chopped

- 1/2 teaspoon ground nutmeg

- 1 cup almond meal

- 4 tablespoons tomato paste

- 1/2 small butternut pumpkin, finely chopped

- 6 asparagus spears, lower ends trimmed and discarded

- 1 handful of activated macadamia nuts, roughly chopped (see Ingredients Glossary)

Preheat the oven to 180°C (350°F).

Line two loaf tins with baking paper.

Place the zucchini, carrot and parsnip in a large bowl and squeeze out the excess water using your hands, then set to one side.

In a food processor pulse the chicken mince, bacon, eggs, chilli, onion, garlic, salt, pepper, parsley, spring onion, nutmeg, almond meal and tomato paste until well combined.

Place the butternut pumpkin in a steamer and cook until tender but firm.

Tip the wet mixture from the food processor into the bowl with the grated vegetables and mix well.

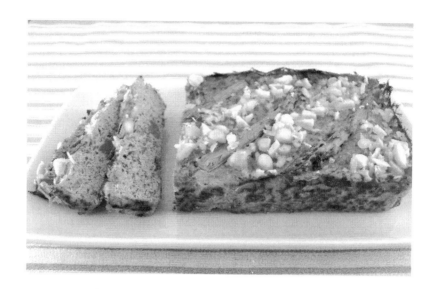

Finely chop one-third of the bottom of each asparagus spear, reserving the rest, and set them aside.

Add the chopped asparagus to the mixture, then stir through the pumpkin.

Divide the mixture between the two loaf tins, press the reserved asparagus into the top of the loaves, sprinkle with the macadamia nuts and bake for 1 hour.

Serve with a mixed salad.

This tasty meatloaf will please everyone. It is great served warm on the day or cut up for lunches during the week. It is also packed with hidden vegetables that no one would ever know about!

Tip: This dish is great as leftovers either cold or hot and can be frozen and reheated later.

Chicken Poached in Stock with Kelp Noodles

SERVES 4–6

Stock

- 4 cups water

- 5cm (2in) piece of fresh ginger, roughly chopped

- 6 cloves garlic, roughly chopped

- 1 large handful of coriander (cilantro), roots trimmed roughly chopped (keep some leaves aside to garnish)

- 1 large carrot, roughly chopped

- 1 long red chilli, seeded and finely chopped

- 1 cinnamon stick

- 4 star anise

- 6 spring onions (scallions), roughly chopped

- juice of 1 lime

- 1 cup coconut aminos or tamari sauce (see Ingredients Glossary for both)

- 1 medium whole chicken, washed

- 1 large carrot, roughly chopped

- 1 bunch of choy sum, roughly chopped

- 1x340g (11 3/4oz) packet of kelp noodles (see Ingredients Glossary)

- 1 spring onion (scallion), finely chopped, to garnish

- 1 long red chilli, seeded and finely sliced, to garnish

- 1 lime, cut into wedges, to serve

First make the stock. In a very large pot, add the water, ginger, garlic, coriander, carrot, chilli, cinnamon, star anise, spring onion, lime juice and coconut aminos and bring to the boil. Add the chicken and top up with water until the chicken is covered. Bring to the boil, reduce to a simmer and cook, covered, for 2 hours. Take the chicken out using tongs and set aside to cool.

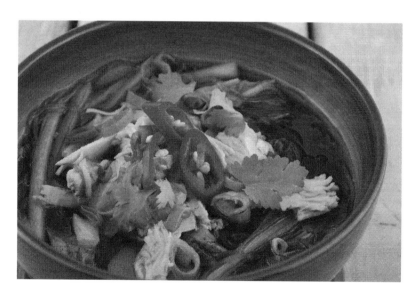

Once cooled, shred the chicken meat and discard the carcass. Strain the stock and place it back on the stove. Add additional water so that the stock is not too salty to taste and skim off any impurities that rise to the surface. Add the carrot and bring to the boil. Once the carrot has softened, add the choy sum and kelp noodles.

Ladle the stock into serving bowls, top with some shredded chicken, spring onion, coriander leaves and chilli, and serve with a wedge of lime.

This makes a lovely, full-flavoured stock, and any of the shredded chicken that you might not use for the dish also works well in the Nori Rolls.

Coconut and Turmeric Chicken Skewers

SERVES 2

- 1 brown onion, roughly chopped

- 3 cloves garlic, roughly chopped

- 6 kaffir lime leaves, centre veins removed

- 1 stalk lemongrass stalk, white part only, bruised and roughly chopped

- 1 teaspoon Chinese five-spice (see Ingredients Glossary)

- 1/2 teaspoon ground turmeric

- 1/2 teaspoon ground mild paprika

- 1/4 teaspoon freshly ground black pepper

- 1/4 teaspoon chilli flakes

- 1 teaspoon raw honey (see Ingredients Glossary)

- 1 tablespoon fish sauce

- 1 tablespoon coconut aminos or tamari sauce (see Ingredients Glossary for both)

- 4 teaspoons coconut cream

- 1 tablespoon coconut oil

- 6 chicken thighs, quartered

- 6 wooden skewers, soaked in water

- 1 handful of coriander (cilantro), to garnish

Blend the onion, garlic, kaffir lime leaves, lemongrass, Chinese five-spice, turmeric, paprika, chilli, honey, fish sauce, coconut aminos, coconut cream and coconut oil together with 1 tablespoon of water in a food processor or blender to make a paste.

Coat the chicken pieces in the paste, cover and refrigerate for 2 hours or overnight.

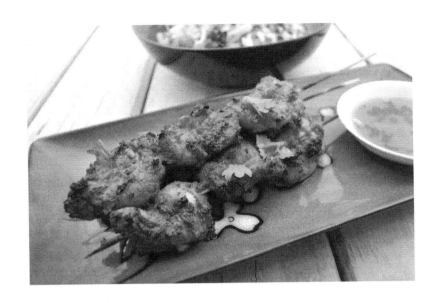

Thread the chicken pieces onto the skewers, then barbecue over an open flame for 5 minutes on each side or until brown and cooked through. Garnish with the coriander and serve the skewers by themselves or with the Cucumber Salad with Vietnamese Herbs (see recipe on above pages).

This is my husband's favourite meal! We cook the skewers outside over some hot coals to give them that real 'hawker meal' flavour—yum!

Tip: These skewers are also great cold the next day.

Sticky Spare Ribs

SERVES 4

- 3 tablespoons tomato paste

- 1/2 cup water

- 1 teaspoon apple cider vinegar

- 3 tablespoons coconut aminos or tamari sauce (see Ingredients Glossary for both)

- 3 cloves garlic, roughly chopped

- 2–3cm (3/4–1 1/4in) piece of fresh ginger, grated

- 1 long red chilli, seeded

- 6–8 medjool dates, pitted (see Ingredients Glossary)

- freshly ground black pepper, to taste

- 1.5kg (3lb 5oz) spare ribs

Blend all the ingredients, except the spare ribs, in a food processor to make a marinade.

Coat the ribs in the marinade, cover and refrigerate for at least 2 hours or, preferably, overnight.

Preheat the oven to 180–190°C (350–375°F).

Bake the ribs on a baking tray lined with baking paper for around 2 hours or until the ribs are nice and sticky and the meat is falling off the bone. Serve immediately.

Perfect for when you are trying to impress a bunch of hungry men—who doesn't love a good sticky spare rib?

Pork or Beef Lemongrass Skewers

SERVES 2

- 2 sticks of lemongrass, white parts only, plus 6 extra lemongrass sticks, to use as skewers

- 4 cloves garlic, roughly chopped

- 1/2 brown onion, roughly chopped

- 1 large red chilli, seeded and finely chopped

- 1 teaspoon coconut sugar (see Ingredients Glossary) or maple syrup

- 1 tablespoon fish sauce

- 1 tablespoon coconut aminos or tamari sauce (see Ingredients Glossary for both)

- freshly ground black pepper, to taste

- 500g (1lb 2oz) pork or beef mince

Lightly crush the 2 white parts of the lemongrass with the flat of a knife, then finely chop.

Mix the lemongrass, garlic, onion, chilli, coconut sugar, fish sauce, coconut aminos and pepper in a blender or food processor to form a paste.

Mix the paste through the mince, cover and refrigerate for at least 2 hours or overnight.

364

Mould the meat over the lemongrass skewers and grill for 2–4 minutes on each side or until cooked through.

Serve with a salad.

Herb and Chilli Chicken

SERVES 2–4

- 1 tablespoon butter or ghee (see Ingredients Glossary)
- 4 chicken Marylands
- 1 teaspoon freshly ground black pepper
- 4 spring onions (scallions), roughly chopped
- 1 small handful of thyme, plus extra, to garnish
- 1 tablespoon raw honey (see Ingredients Glossary)
- 1 tablespoon apple cider vinegar
- pinch of allspice
- 3 cloves garlic, roughly chopped
- 1 long red chilli, seeded and roughly chopped
- pink Himalayan salt, to taste (see Ingredients Glossary)
- freshly ground black pepper, to taste
- 2 handfuls of grape tomatoes

- 1 large zucchini (courgette), roughly chopped

- 1/2 small butternut pumpkin, cubed

- 1 small handful of baby basil leaves

Preheat the oven to 180°C (350°F).

Melt the butter in a pan over a medium heat.

Season the chicken by rubbing pepper into the skin, then cook each Maryland skin-side down in the pan for a few minutes or until the skin is golden brown.

In a blender or food processor, combine the spring onion, thyme, honey, apple cider vinegar, allspice, garlic, chilli, salt and pepper.

Place the chicken skin-side up in a heavy-based casserole dish. Scatter the tomatoes, zucchini and butternut pumpkin around the chicken, pour over the blended mixture and bake for 1 hour or until the juices of the chicken run clear.

Serve topped with the extra thyme and baby basil leaves.

A hearty winter warmer! It is quick to put together and great reheated the next day.

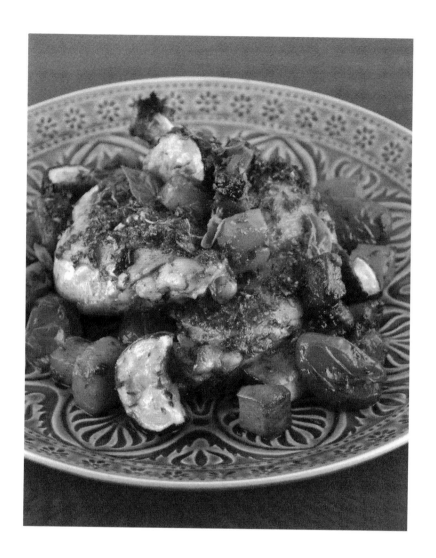

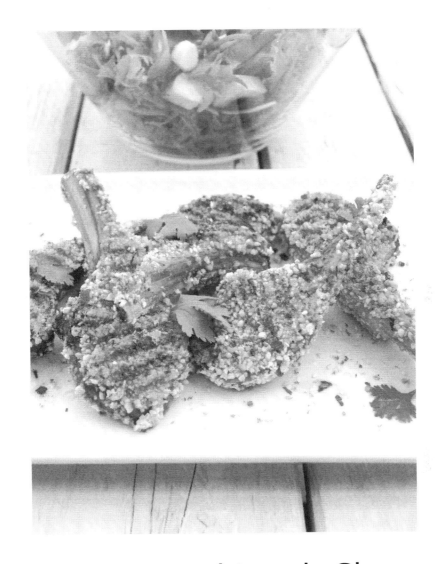

Cashew-encrusted Lamb Chops

SERVES 2–3

- 1 cup unsalted activated cashews (see Ingredients Glossary)

- 1 tablespoon sesame seeds, toasted

- 1/4 teaspoon dried chilli flakes

- zest of 1 lime

- freshly ground black pepper, to taste

- 1 egg

- 6–8 small lamb chops

- 1 handful of coriander (cilantro), roughly chopped

- juice of 1/2 lime

In a food processor or blender, mix the cashews, sesame seeds, chilli flakes, lime zest and pepper until you have fairly fine crumbs. Transfer the mixture to a bowl and set aside.

Whisk the egg with a fork to make an egg wash.

Dip the chops in the egg wash and then the crust mix, making sure the chops are well coated.

Heat a griddle pan over a medium to high heat and cook the chops for 5 minutes on each side. Remove from the heat, cover with foil and rest for 5 minutes.

Top with coriander and a squeeze of lime juice and serve with a salad.

The zestiness of the lime works so well with the other flavours in this crust. These chops are always a crowd pleaser at BBQs. They are also super tasty cold the next day.

Kangaroo Steak with a Red Wine and Peppercorn Sauce

SERVES 2

- 2 kangaroo steaks
- coconut oil or ghee (see Ingredients Glossary), for coating
- freshly ground black pepper, to taste
- Red Wine and Peppercorn Sauce, to serve (see recipe on above pages)
- roasted vegetables of your choice (sweet potato, pumpkin, cauliflower, carrot)
- 1 small handful of flat-leaf (Italian) parsley, to garnish

Rub each steak with coconut oil and season with pepper.

Place a grill pan over a high heat and cook the kangaroo on one side until the moisture just shows, then repeat on the other side. Place the steaks on a chopping board, cover with foil and rest for 10 minutes.

Place each steak on a plate and pour over the Red Wine and Peppercorn Sauce. Garnish with parsley leaves.

370

Serve with roasted vegetables.

> Kangaroo is a great lean meat, packed with nutrients. If you have never tried it, this dish is a great introduction!

Tip: If you can't find kangaroo, this recipe works just as well with 2 porterhouse steaks.

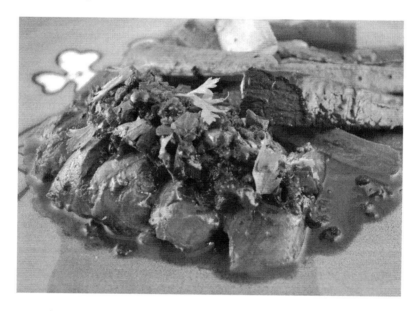

Meatballs in Bolognese Sauce

SERVES 6

- 500g (1lb 2oz) pork mince
- 500g (1lb 2oz) beef mince
- 2–3 cloves garlic, roughly chopped
- 3 bacon rashers, roughly chopped

- 1 large handful of flat-leaf (Italian) parsley, plus extra to serve

- 10 basil leaves

- pink Himalayan salt, to taste (see Ingredients Glossary)

- freshly ground black pepper, to taste

- 2 eggs

- 1 quantity of Bolognese Sauce (see recipe on above pages)

- 3 large carrots, julienned

- 3 large zucchini (courgettes), julienned

Preheat the oven to 180°C (350°F).

Using your hands, combine the pork and beef mince in a large bowl.

Place the mince, garlic, bacon, parsley, basil, salt, pepper and eggs in a food processor and blend until well combined.

Roll the mixture into golf ball-sized portions and place in a large ceramic cooking dish, making sure they are spaced at least 1cm (1/2in) apart. Pour over the Bolognese Sauce, making sure all the meatballs are covered, then cook in the oven for 30 minutes.

Just before the meatballs are ready to come out, place the carrot and zucchini in a large bowl and cover with boiling water for 5 minutes or until they are soft, then drain.

Arrange the carrot and zucchini on serving plates and cover with the meatballs and sauce. Garnish with the extra parsley and serve.

I love making a big batch of these meatballs and freezing them for when we do not feel like cooking on a busy weeknight. The meatballs are so tasty and this recipe is just bursting with vitamins, minerals and anti-oxidants!

Tip: The meatballs and sauce can be frozen before cooking and prepared at a later date.

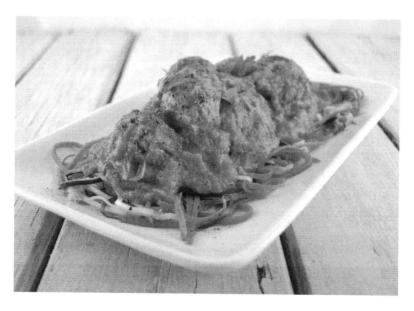

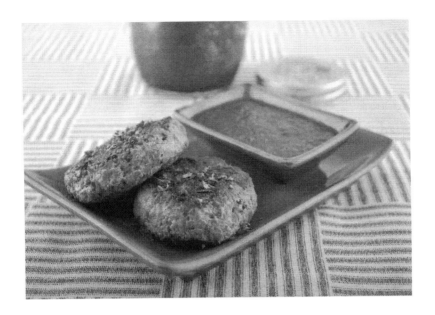

Pork Patties

MAKES 8–12

- 1 large brown onion, roughly chopped
- 3 cloves garlic, finely chopped
- 1 long red chilli, seeded and finely chopped
- 1 medium carrot, grated
- 1 small handful of flat-leaf (Italian) parsley, roughly chopped
- 2 heaped tablespoons wholegrain mustard
- 1 tablespoon tomato paste
- 1 tablespoon raw honey (see Ingredients Glossary)
- 1 egg

- pink Himalayan salt, to taste (see Ingredients Glossary)

- freshly ground black pepper, to taste

- 500g (1lb 2oz) pork mince

- butter or ghee (see Ingredients Glossary), for frying

Blend all the ingredients, except the butter, in a food processor until the mixture is quite wet.

Melt the butter in a pan over a medium heat. Using wet hands, form meat patties about the size of your palm, then place them in the pan and cook until they are golden brown on both sides.

Serve with your favourite salad and mayonnaise, or with tomato sauce (see recipe on above pages).

> The wholegrain mustard and honey gives these pork patties a lovely tangy flavour with a touch of sweetness.

Tip: These can also be enjoyed cold as a delicious snack.

Slow-cooked Osso Bucco

SERVES 4

- 4 beef osso bucco

- pink Himalayan salt, to taste (see Ingredients Glossary)

- freshly ground black pepper, to taste, plus 1/2 teaspoon extra

- 3 tablespoons butter or ghee (see Ingredients Glossary)

- 2 medium brown onions, roughly chopped

- 4 cloves garlic, finely chopped

- 2 large carrots, roughly chopped

- 4 sticks celery, roughly chopped

- 2 tablespoons tomato paste

- 2 cups Bone Broth (see recipe on above pages)

- 1/2 cup good white wine

- 2x400g (14oz) tins whole tomatoes

- 2 bay leaves

- 4 sprigs thyme

- 1 quantity of Sweet Potato Mash (see recipe on above pages)

- 1 handful of flat-leaf (Italian) parsley, to garnish

Season the osso bucco with salt and pepper.

Melt 1 tablespoon of the butter in a large pan over a high heat and brown the osso bucco on both sides. Set to one side.

In a large heavy-based pot over a medium heat, melt the remaining butter, then add the onion, garlic, carrot and celery and sauté until the onion is soft. Add the tomato paste, Bone Broth, white wine, tinned tomatoes, bay leaves, thyme and extra black pepper. Bring to the boil, then reduce to a very low heat. Add the osso bucco, making sure it is submerged in the liquid and cook, covered, for 2–3 hours or until the meat is falling off the bone.

Serve on a bed of Sweet Potato Mash and garnish with parsley leaves.

Slow cooking is a great way to use cheaper, tougher cuts of meat. This recipe is equally as tasty if you want to replace the white wine with additional bone broth.

The Best Steak and Chips

SERVES 2

- 2 porterhouse steaks, left at room temperature for 20 minutes

- small amount of coconut oil, for rubbing

- pink Himalayan salt, to taste (see Ingredients Glossary)

- freshly ground black pepper, to taste

- 3 tablespoons coconut oil

- 4 large parsnips, cut into batons

Rub the steaks with coconut oil and season with salt and pepper. Cook the steaks to your liking, then rest them on a chopping board, covered with foil, for 10 minutes.

While the steaks are resting, heat the 3 tablespoons of coconut oil in a pan over a high heat and shallow-fry the parsnip batons until golden brown. Using tongs, place the parsnips on some paper towel to drain any excess oil. Season with salt and pepper.

Serve the steaks with the parsnip chips and your favourite salad.

This recipe is a MUST! Wait until you try the parsnip chips in coconut oil—you'll be hooked.

Steak with Spinach Cream and Roasted Tomato

SERVES 4

Roasted Tomato

- 14 grape tomatoes, halved

- 2 cloves garlic, minced

- pink Himalayan salt, to taste (see Ingredients Glossary)

- freshly ground black pepper, to taste

Spinach Cream

- 1 teaspoon butter or ghee (see Ingredients Glossary)

- 2 cloves garlic, roughly chopped

- 1 brown onion, finely chopped

- 1/4 cup vegetable stock

- 1/4 cup coconut cream

- 2–3 handfuls of baby spinach leaves, roughly chopped

- pinch of ground nutmeg

- freshly ground black pepper, to taste

- 4 beef steaks, left at room temperature for 20–30 minutes

- 2 zucchini (courgettes), peeled into strips using a julienne peeler

- 2 tablespoons nutritional yeast, to serve (see Ingredients Glossary)

- 1 handful of flat-leaf (Italian) parsley

Preheat the oven to 180°C (350°F).

First make the roasted tomato. Scatter the tomatoes on a baking tray lined with baking paper and season with the minced garlic, salt and pepper and roast for 15–20 minutes. Set aside.

To make the spinach cream, melt the butter in a small saucepan over a medium heat. Add the garlic and onion and sauté until soft. Add the stock and coconut cream and bring to the boil, then add the spinach and simmer for 5 minutes. Blend the soup until you have a smooth consistency, then add the nutmeg and pepper and stir through. Adjust the seasoning and add more stock if the soup is too thick.

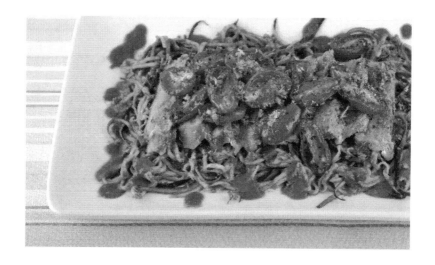

Cook the steak to your liking, then rest the steak on a chopping board, covered with foil, for 10 minutes.

While the steak is resting, place the zucchini in a bowl and cover with boiling water for approximately 5 minutes or until soft. Drain the zucchini and combine with the spinach cream.

Plate the spinach cream zucchini and top with sliced steak and roasted tomatoes. Serve with a sprinkling of nutritional yeast and parsley leaves.

This makes an impressive meal and is great to serve on a large sharing plate if you are making it for dinner guests. The nutritional yeast gives it that little kick—like Parmesan cheese would.

Tip: A rare to medium-rare steak has the best nutritional value.

Occasional Treats and Desserts

Banana Bread

SERVES 8

- butter or ghee (see Ingredients Glossary), for greasing
- 6 eggs
- 2 tablespoons coconut oil
- 2 tablespoons coconut cream
- 1 teaspoon vanilla bean paste (see Ingredients Glossary)
- 3 large ripe bananas, mashed
- 2 cups almond meal
- 1 teaspoon baking powder
- 1/2 teaspoon ground cinnamon
- pinch of ground nutmeg
- 1 handful of activated pumpkin seeds (pepitas)

This banana bread will be a hit with everyone—Paleo or not! It is best served warm, but that usually isn't a problem as it is generally gone within half an hour!

Preheat the oven to 180°C (350°F).

Line a loaf tin with baking paper and grease with butter.

Beat the eggs, coconut oil, coconut cream, vanilla bean paste and bananas until well combined.

Place the almond meal, baking powder, cinnamon and nutmeg in a large bowl and mix until well combined.

Add the dry mixture to the wet mixture and stir until well combined. Pour into the loaf tin, sprinkle with the pumpkin seeds and bake for 50–55 minutes or until the loaf springs back when touched in the centre.

Frozen Fruit Icy Pops

MAKES 6

- 1 cup raspberries
- 1 tablespoon filtered water
- set of six ice-cream moulds
- 3 kiwifruit, peeled

Blend the raspberries and filtered water to a smooth consistency using a hand blender and fill the ice-cream moulds to halfway with the mixture.

Blend the kiwifruit (they contain enough of their own liquid) with a hand blender and fill the moulds to the top with the mixture.

Place the moulds in the freezer and serve once frozen.

Tip: Placing the icy pops under warm running water can help to remove them from the moulds when they are stuck.

Having trouble getting the kids to eat fruit? Blend it up and make it look like an icy pop—problem solved!

Raspberry and Rosewater Ice-cream Pops

MAKES 6

- 2 cups raspberries
- 2 tablespoons filtered water
- set of six ice-cream moulds
- 1/2 cup coconut cream
- 1/2 teaspoon rosewater (see Ingredients Glossary)

384

Blend the raspberries and filtered water to a smooth consistency using a hand blender, then place a teaspoon of the mixture in the bottom of each mould.

Add the coconut cream and rosewater to the remaining raspberry mixture and combine. Top up the moulds with the blended mixture and freeze.

> Prepare these for the kids and they won't be asking for store-bought ice creams anymore! They contain no added sugar and the raspberries are full of anti-oxidant goodness!

Tip: Placing the pops under warm running water can help to remove them from the moulds when they are stuck.

Blueberry Ice Cream

SERVES 2

- 1/3 cup cold coconut cream (from the fridge)
- 1 cup frozen blueberries
- 1 teaspoon vanilla bean paste (see Ingredients Glossary)
- coconut flakes, toasted, to garnish

Place the coconut cream, blueberries and vanilla bean paste in a blender and purée until smooth. Serve topped with toasted coconut flakes and enjoy.

This ice cream takes 2 minutes to make and it's so tasty!

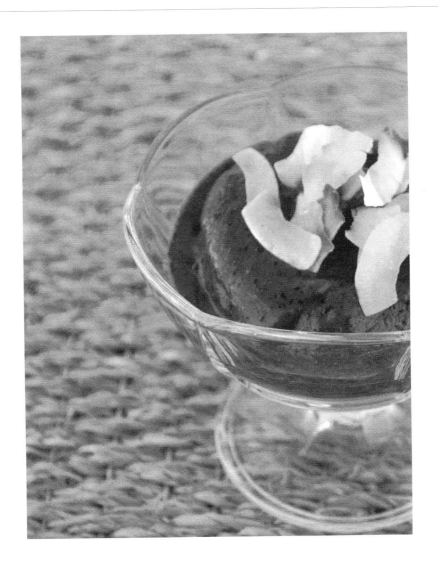

Chocolate Cherry Bites

MAKES ABOUT 25

- 34 cherries, cut in half and pitted

- 2 cups toasted shredded coconut

- 2 tablespoons coconut oil

- 70g (2 1/2oz) cacao butter (see Ingredients Glossary)

- 1 cup coconut cream

- 1 teaspoon vanilla bean paste (see Ingredients Glossary)

- 200g (7oz) dark chocolate (at least 85% cacao)

- 1 small handful of cacao nibs (see Ingredients Glossary)

Preheat the oven to 160°C (320°F).

Line both a baking tray and a baking tin (approximately 18cmx28cmx3cm deep/7inx11 1/4inx1 1/4in deep) with baking paper.

Place the cherries on the tray and roast for 20 minutes. Set the cherries aside to cool slightly then place them in a blender with 1 cup of the shredded coconut and the coconut oil and blend until well combined. Press the cherry mixture firmly into the base of the baking tin and freeze for 5–10 minutes.

Place the cacao butter, coconut cream and vanilla bean paste in a saucepan over a gentle heat and stir until the cacao butter has melted. Mix the remaining shredded coconut with the cacao butter mixture and pour it over the first cherry layer, again pressing down firmly. Place the tray back in the freezer for another 5–10 minutes.

Over a double boiler, melt the dark chocolate, then pour it over the slice as the top layer. Sprinkle over the cacao nibs and place the tray back in the freezer until set.

Cut the slice into bite-sized pieces and store in the fridge.

I make these over Christmas when cherries are in season; they are HEAVENLY!

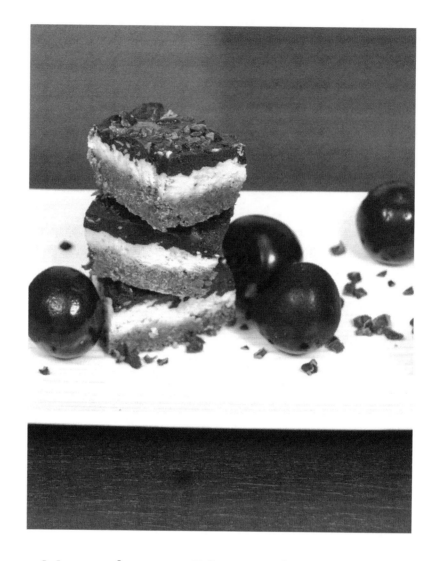

Coffee Hazelnut Chocolate Balls

MAKES 10

- 2 tablespoons cacao butter (see Ingredients Glossary)

- 1/2 cup activated hazelnuts (see Ingredients Glossary)

- 6 medjool dates, pitted and roughly chopped (see Ingredients Glossary)

- 2 teaspoons raw cacao powder (see Ingredients Glossary)

- 6 teaspoons espresso coffee

- 2 tablespoons activated pumpkin seeds (pepitas) (see Ingredients Glossary)

- 1/2 cup cacao nibs (see Ingredients Glossary)

Melt the cacao butter in a saucepan over a gentle heat.

Place the melted cacao butter with the hazelnuts, medjool dates, cacaco powder, coffee and pumpkin seeds in a blender and pulse until the mixture comes together.

Using your hands, roll the mixture into bite-sized balls, then coat them in the cacao nibs. Place the balls in the fridge to chill before serving.

Store in an airtight container in the fridge and use as required.

These little balls of coffee and chocolate goodness make the perfect, sophisticated adult dessert or treat.

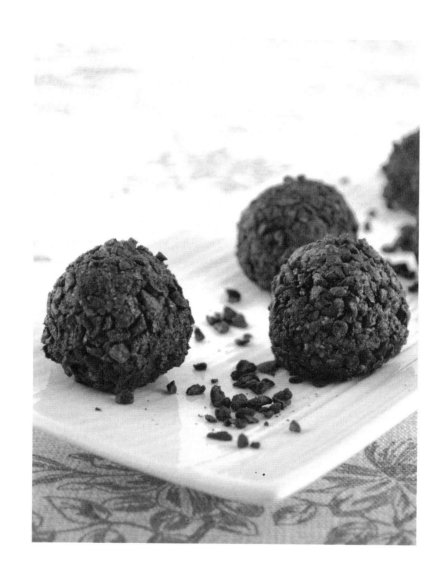

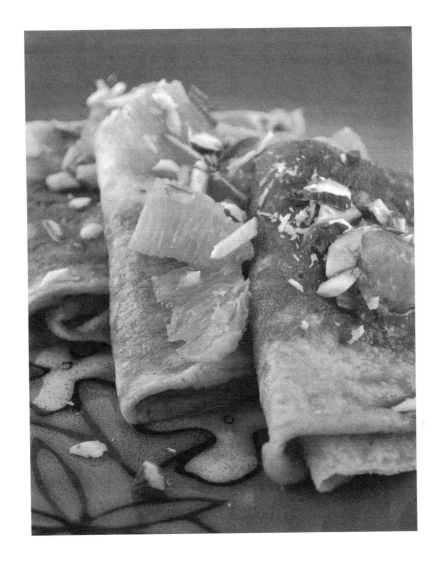

Banana Pancakes

MAKES 6–8 LARGE PANCAKES

- 1/2 cup tapioca flour
- 1 tablespoon baking powder
- 1 tablespoon coconut flour
- pinch of pink Himalayan salt

- 4 eggs

- 2/3 cup almond milk (see recipe on above pages)

- 1/4 teaspoon vanilla bean paste (see Ingredients Glossary)

- 2 tablespoons butter or ghee (see Ingredients Glossary), melted, plus extra, for cooking

- 4 small ripe bananas, mashed with a fork

Place the tapioca flour, baking powder, coconut flour and salt in a bowl and mix until combined. Add the eggs, almond milk, vanilla bean paste, butter and bananas, whisking continuously until the batter is combined and aerated.

Melt a little butter in a frying pan over a medium heat. Add a small ladle of the batter to the pan and cook until bubbles appear on the surface and the pancake is golden underneath. Flip the pancake and cook for a further minute or until that side is golden as well. Repeat until all the remaining batter has been used. Serve immediately.

Before we changed to Paleo, I had a favourite pancake recipe that I used to make for my husband. Coming up with a good Paleo version eluded me for years. I could never win him over because he always compared them to the ones containing gluten. But I came up with a winner with these ones—and he LOVES them!

Serving suggestions: Serve with double cream or coconut cream, orange segments and chopped almonds, drizzled with maple syrup.

Mango, Ginger and Lime Sorbet

SERVES 2

- 3 tablespoons coconut cream

- 2cm (3/4in) piece of fresh ginger, grated

- juice and zest of 2 limes, plus extra, to serve

- 1 mango, seeded and roughly chopped

Stir the coconut cream and ginger together in a saucepan over a low heat for 5 minutes, allowing the flavours to infuse. Take the pan off the heat and allow to cool.

Place the cooled coconut cream and ginger, lime zest and juice and the mango in a blender and mix until well combined.

Pour the mixture into a stainless steel bowl and place in the freezer, briskly whisking the sorbet every 20 minutes to prevent crystallisation. Repeat this process until you have the desired consistency (this takes approximately 90 minutes).

Serve with a little zest on top.

This recipe takes a bit of elbow grease (if you don't have an ice-cream maker), but it's worth it in the end. Tangy, sweet goodness!

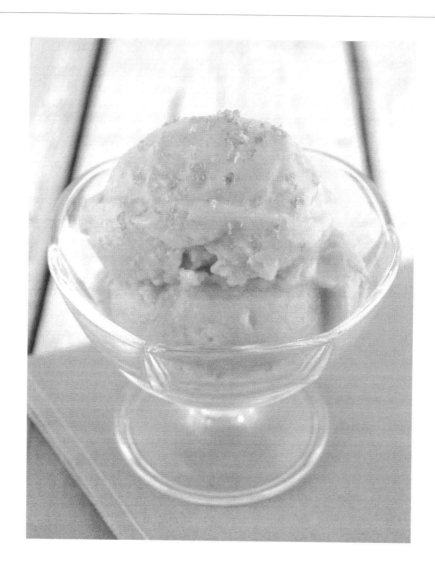

Fruit and Nut Chocolate

MAKES ONE 18CM X 28CM (7IN X 11 1/4IN) BAR

- 1/3 cup activated pumpkin seeds (pepitas), roughly chopped (see Ingredients Glossary)

- 1 handful of dried apricots, roughly chopped (sulphur free)

- 1/2 cup activated macadamia nuts, roughly chopped (see Ingredients Glossary)

- 1/4 cup coconut oil

- 2 tablespoons coconut sugar, or any other natural sweetener (see Ingredients Glossary)

- 2 tablespoons cacao butter (see Ingredients Glossary)

- 1/2 cup raw cacao powder (see Ingredients Glossary)

Line an 18cmx28cmx3cm (7inx11 1/4inx1 1/4in) baking tin with baking paper making sure the paper is up over the edges. Scatter the pumpkin seeds, dried apricots and macadamia nuts on the tray and set aside.

Over a double boiler, melt the coconut oil, coconut sugar and cacao butter together, then add the cacao powder to the oil and mix until well combined. Tip

396

the chocolate mix over the fruit and nuts, making sure to coat them all. Place the tray in the freezer until set.

Break the chocolate into pieces and store in the fridge or freezer. Serve cold.

This chocolate is simple to make, has a good crunch factor and really hits the spot when you need a sweet treat! Make sure you look out for dried apricots that are sulphur free. They won't look as pretty, but they are much better for you.

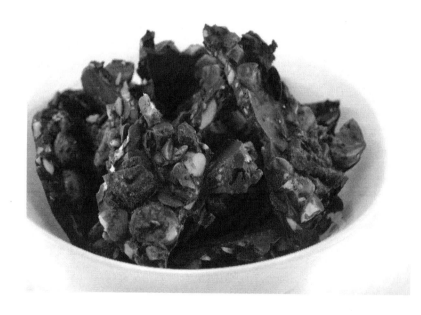

Peach and Pear Fruit Leather

MAKES 2

- 2 peaches, roughly chopped
- 4 small pears, cored and roughly chopped
- juice of 1/2 lemon

Place the peaches and pears in a saucepan over a low to medium heat. Squeeze the lemon juice into the pan and cook until the fruit starts to break down, stirring continuously. Once the fruit has softened, set aside to cool.

Once the fruit is cool, blend to a smooth consistency.

If dehydrating in an oven, pour the mixture evenly onto a baking tray lined with plastic wrap to a 2mm (1/16in) thickness and dehydrate at your oven's lowest temperature (70–100°C/150–200°F) with the door slightly ajar. The fruit mixture should dry in 6–10 hours. Frequently test if the leather is done (it will be ready when it turns slightly translucent and can be peeled from the tray). You can test for dryness by gently pressing the leather in different places—it should be slightly tacky but not sticky and no indents should be evident.

If using a dehydrator, spread your mixture on the trays provided and dehydrate according to the manual.

> Tasty and simple to make and better than anything store bought. No hidden preservatives and additives!

Ginger Nut Cookies

MAKES 16–20

- 3 cups almond meal
- 2 tablespoons ground ginger
- 2 teaspoons ground cinnamon
- 1 teaspoon ground nutmeg
- 1/2 teaspoon ground cloves
- 1 teaspoon baking powder
- 1/3 cup coconut sugar (see Ingredients Glossary)
- 4 tablespoons coconut oil
- 1/4 cup maple syrup

Preheat the oven to 170°C (325°F).

Line a large baking tray with baking paper. In a large bowl, mix the almond meal, ginger, cinnamon, nutmeg, cloves and baking powder together until well combined.

Melt the coconut sugar, coconut oil and maple syrup in a saucepan over a medium heat, stirring continuously until the coconut sugar has dissolved and the liquid starts to foam. Quickly pour the mixture into the dry ingredients and mix with a spoon until well combined. The mixture will be moist and a little crumbly.

Take a dessertspoon-sized portion of the mixture and gently roll it into a little ball, flattening it between your palms before placing it on the baking tray. Repeat with the rest of the mixture, leaving a little space between the cookies (don't worry if they are a little cracked, this is part of the look).

Bake the cookies for 15–20 minutes, turning the tray around halfway to ensure even cooking. Allow to cool for a few minutes on the tray before transferring to a wire rack to cool completely. They will harden as they cool down.

Once you have made these, hide them or they won't last long!

Raspberry and Cream Biscuits

MAKES 10–12

- 1 egg
- 1/4 cup coconut oil
- 1 teaspoon vanilla bean paste (see Ingredients Glossary)
- 1/4 cup raw honey (see Ingredients Glossary)

- 1 1/4 cups almond meal

- 2 tablespoons coconut flour

- 1/4 teaspoon baking powder

- 1/4 cup arrowroot powder

- 1/4 cup desiccated coconut

- 1 teaspoon gelatine

- 1 cup raspberries

- 1/4 cup coconut cream

- 1/4 cup coconut butter

- 1/2 teaspoon maple syrup

Preheat the oven to 170°C (325°F).

Line a baking tray with baking paper.

Whisk the egg, coconut oil, vanilla bean paste and honey together in a bowl until well combined.

In a separate bowl, mix the almond meal, coconut flour, baking powder, arrowroot powder and desiccated coconut, making sure it is well combined.

Combine the wet and dry ingredients—the mixture will be a little sticky. Take teaspoonfuls of the mixture, roll into small bite-sized balls and place on the baking tray. Press them with a fork to flatten then bake for 20 minutes. Cool on a wire rack.

While the biscuits are baking, soften the gelatine in a small amount of water, then blend with the raspberries in a blender. Place in the fridge to set.

Place the coconut cream, coconut butter and maple syrup in a blender and mix until thick and creamy, then place in the fridge to chill.

Remove the raspberry mixture from the fridge and whisk with a fork until you have the consistency of thick raspberry jam.

To assemble, sandwich a teaspoon of jam and a teaspoon of coconut cream between two biscuits.

Store in an airtight container in the fridge.

Who loves Monte Carlo biscuits? Well, if you do, you will love these little beauties!

Orange and Poppy Seed Cupcakes

MAKES 24 MINI OR 9 LARGE CUPCAKES

- 1 cup coconut milk
- 1/3 cup coconut sugar (see Ingredients Glossary)
- zest of 1 orange, plus extra, to garnish
- 6 eggs

- 2 egg whites

- 2 tablespoons coconut oil

- 2 teaspoons vanilla extract

- 1/2 teaspoon baking power

- 1/2 cup coconut flour

- 1/4 cup tapioca flour

- 1 tablespoon poppy seeds

- cacao nibs, to garnish (see Ingredients Glossary)

Cashew Cream
- 2 cups cashews, soaked overnight in water and drained

- 2 teaspoons vanilla bean paste (see Ingredients Glossary)

- 1 tablespoon coconut oil

- 2 tablespoons maple syrup

Chocolate Orange Cream
- 2 small avocados

- 2 tablespoons maple syrup

- 6–7 drops orange extract

- 1 tablespoon orange juice

- 2 tablespoons raw cacao powder (see Ingredients Glossary)

- 1 tablespoon cacao butter (see Ingredients Glossary)

Preheat the oven to 180°C (350°F).

Line two 12-cup mini muffin tins with mini patty cases.

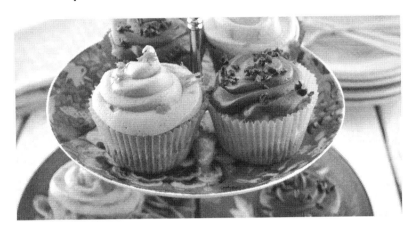

In a small saucepan over a low heat, combine the coconut milk, coconut sugar and orange zest and warm until the sugar has dissolved and the flavours have infused.

Beat the eggs and egg whites together in the bowl of an electric mixer until light and aerated. Slowly add the coconut oil and vanilla extract, then the baking powder, coconut flour and tapioca flour and mix until just combined. Remove the bowl from the mixer, stir through the warm coconut milk mixture and the poppy seeds and divide the mixture evenly between the patty cases.

Bake for 25 minutes or until a skewer inserted into the middle comes out clean. Turn out onto a wire rack to cool.

While the cupcakes are cooking, make the cashew cream and chocolate orange cream. Blend the ingredients of each cream together and place in the fridge to chill.

Once the cupcakes are cool, pipe the cashew cream on half of the cupcakes and garnish with the extra orange zest, and pipe the chocolate orange cream on the remaining cupcakes and sprinkle with cacao nibs.

> These are best eaten the same day, which usually isn't a problem! I have provided two delicious icings to top the cupcakes with—a cashew cream and a chocolate orange cream.

Coconut and Mango Chia Seed Pudding

SERVES 2

- 1 cup of Paleo Granola (see recipe on above pages)

- 1 quantity of Chia Seed Pudding (see recipe below—remember it needs to be prepared the night before)

- 1 mango, seeded and diced

Place layers of the Paleo Granola, Chia Seed Pudding and mango in two serving glasses and serve.

This is the perfect summer treat—enjoy!

Chia Seed Pudding

SERVES 2

- 1/2 cup coconut milk

- 1/2 cup almond milk (see recipe on above pages)

- 1 teaspoon vanilla bean paste (see Ingredients Glossary)

- 2 tablespoons chia seeds (see Ingredients Glossary)

Place the coconut milk, almond milk, vanilla bean paste and chia seeds in a bowl and mix until well combined. Cover and refrigerate overnight.

This basic chia pudding is a great base for a breakfast or dessert—just add your favourite fruit and nut combinations. The chia seeds swell to make a lovely thick vanilla pudding. Add some coconut cream to make it extra creamy.

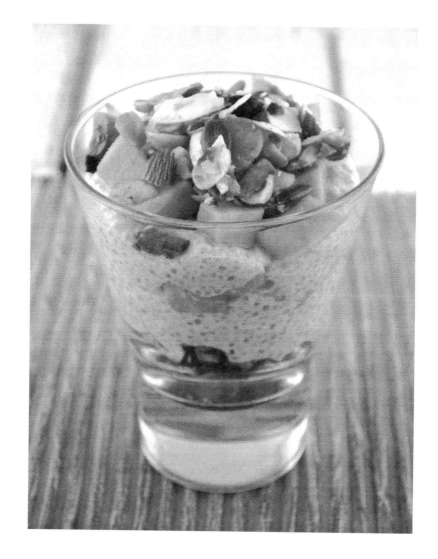

Jaffa Cups

MAKES 10–12 MINI CUPS

- 2 tablespoons coconut butter
- 2 tablespoons coconut milk
- 1 tablespoon raw honey (see Ingredients Glossary)
- 5–7 drops of orange extract

- 2 tablespoons cacao butter (see Ingredients Glossary)

- 1/2 cup raw cacao powder (see Ingredients Glossary)

- 1/4 cup coconut oil

- 3–5 drops stevia, depending on desired sweetness (you still want a strong dark chocolate flavour)

- zest of 1 orange

- 1/4 cup cacao nibs, to garnish (see Ingredients Glossary)

Place 10–12 mini patty pans on a baking tray.

Place the coconut butter, coconut milk, honey and orange extract in a blender and mix until combined. Pour into a bowl and place in the fridge to chill.

In a double boiler over a low heat, gently melt the cacao butter, cacao powder, coconut oil, stevia and orange zest. Once melted, turn off the heat and leave the bowl over the water to stay warm.

Place a teaspoon of the orange chocolate mixture in each of the mini patty pans and place in the freezer for 10 minutes—leaving the remaining mixture on the double boiler to stay warm.

Take out the tray of patty pans and add a teaspoon of the coconut cream mix to each, then place it back in the freezer for 5 minutes. Take out the tray of patty pans again and evenly divide the remaining orange chocolate mixture between them. Sprinkle each chocolate cup with cacao nibs and place back in the freezer until set. Serve cold.

The creamy coconut–orange middle oozes from the middle of these cups when you bite into them. Yummy, orangey, chocolatey goodness!

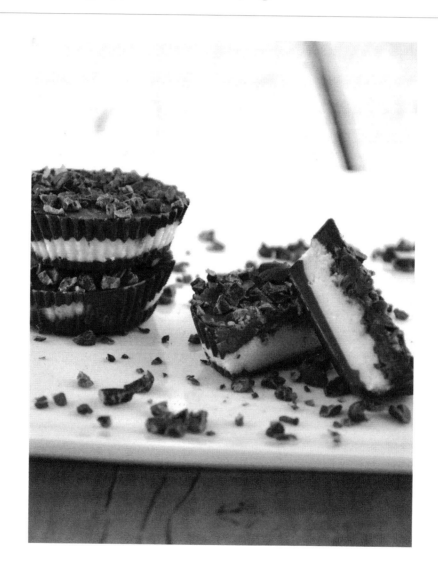

Lime, Coconut and Pandanus Panna Cotta

MAKES 3

- 1 teaspoon gelatine
- 2 tablespoons boiling filtered water
- 2/3 cup coconut cream
- 1/2 cup almond milk (see recipe on above pages)
- 6 pandanus leaves, roughly chopped (see Ingredients Glossary)
- 1 tablespoon raw honey (see Ingredients Glossary)
- zest of 1 lime

Place the gelatine in the boiling filtered water to soften. Set aside.

Place the coconut cream, almond milk, pandanus and honey in a food processor or blender and mix until combined. Pour the mixture into a saucepan and bring to the boil, then reduce the heat and a simmer for 5 minutes. Turn off the heat and allow the mixture to sit for 10 minutes letting the flavours infuse. Strain the liquid and place it back on the stove in the saucepan.

Over a medium heat add the softened gelatine and cook until it all dissolves. Add the lime zest then pour

410

the mixture into panna cotta cups or ramekins and place in the fridge to set (at least 4 hours, preferably overnight). Serve cold.

I got the inspiration for this recipe from a panna cotta recipe I saw in one of Luke Nguyen's cookbooks. The pandanus leaves add an almost vanilla-like flavour to the dish.

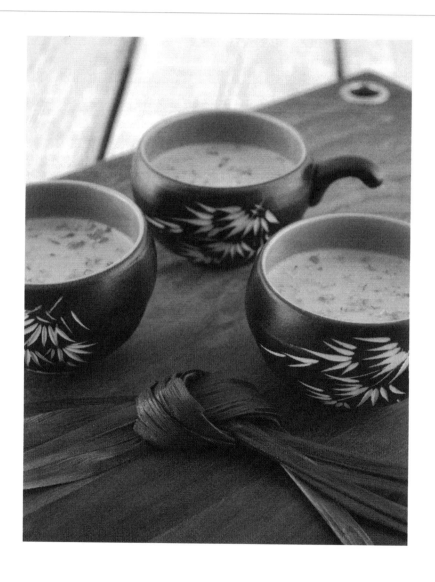

Rhubarb, Blueberry and Apple Crumble

SERVES 6–8

Fruit Mix

- 4 sticks rhubarb, cut into 2cm (3/4in) pieces
- 1 tablespoon coconut sugar (see Ingredients Glossary) or maple syrup (omit if you prefer a more tart flavour)
- juice of 1/2 lemon
- 4 granny smith apples, peeled, cored and roughly chopped
- 1 cup blueberries (you can use frozen)

Crumble

- 1 cup activated almonds, roughly chopped (see Ingredients Glossary)
- 1/4 cup coconut flakes
- 1 tablespoon coconut sugar (see Ingredients Glossary)
- 1 teaspoon ground cinnamon
- 1 teaspoon vanilla bean paste (see Ingredients Glossary)
- 2 teaspoons coconut oil

Preheat the oven to 170°C (325°F).

First make the fruit mix. Place the rhubarb, coconut sugar and lemon juice in a saucepan and cook over a low heat for 10–15 minutes or until the rhubarb starts to break down. Add the apples and cook for a further 10 minutes. Add the blueberries and stir through. Spoon the mixture into ramekins.

Next make the crumble. Place the almonds, coconut flakes, coconut sugar, cinnamon, vanilla bean paste and coconut oil in a food processor or blender and pulse until you get a nice crumbly mixture. Sprinkle the crumble over the top of each ramekin and bake for 25 minutes.

I love the addition of blueberries to the classic combination of apple and rhubarb. The blueberries just add a lovely 'pop' in your mouth when you eat this crumble.

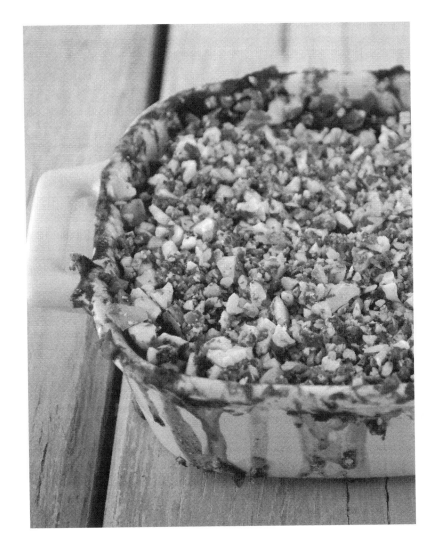

Rosewater Chocolate Mousse with Raspberry Coulis

SERVES 2–4

Cashew Cream
- 2 cups cashews, soaked in water overnight and drained

- 3 teaspoons vanilla bean paste (see Ingredients Glossary)

- 2 tablespoons maple syrup

- up to 1/4 cup filtered water

Chocolate Mousse
- 2 avocados, halved, stones removed

- 2 tablespoons raw cacao powder (see Ingredients Glossary)

- 1/2 teaspoon rosewater (see Ingredients Glossary)

- 2 tablespoons maple syrup

Raspberry Coulis
- 1/2 cup raspberries

- 1/2 cup whole raspberries, to serve

- 3 tablespoons activated pistachios, roughly chopped, plus extra, to serve (see Ingredients Glossary)

First make the cashew cream. Place the cashews, vanilla bean paste, maple syrup and half of the filtered water in a blender and pulse until combined (adding more water as required until you have a creamy smooth consistency). Transfer to a bowl and chill in the fridge while you make the mousse.

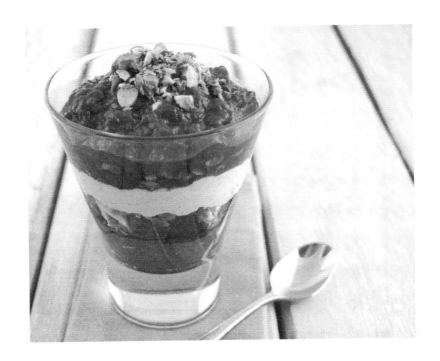

Next make the chocolate mousse. Blend all the mousse ingredients in a food processor or an electric mixer until you have a creamy mousse-like consistency. Transfer to a bowl and chill in the fridge while you make the coulis.

To make the raspberry coulis, place the raspberries in a small saucepan over a low heat and cook until they begin to break down. Take off the heat and allow to cool.

Build the rosewater chocolate mousse layers in a tall glass in the following order: chocolate mousse, whole raspberries and pistachios and the cashew cream. Repeat the layers if necessary. Top with the raspberry coulis and the extra pistachios and chill before serving.

Yum, yum, yum! You would never know that this mousse is dairy-free and packed with avocado. Serve it and have them guessing what the ingredients are! If you want a more chocolatey flavour, add an extra teaspoon of raw cacao powder to the mousse.

Sticky Date Pudding

SERVES 2

Pudding

- butter or ghee (see Ingredients Glossary), for greasing

- 6 medjool dates, pitted and roughly chopped (see Ingredients Glossary)

- 5 tablespoons filtered water

- 1 teaspoon coconut flour

- 1 egg

- 1 ripe banana, peeled

- 1 teaspoon vanilla bean paste (see Ingredients Glossary)

- 1/4 teaspoon baking powder

Sticky Date Syrup

- 2 tablespoons filtered water

- 2 medjool dates, pitted and roughly chopped (see Ingredients Glossary)

- 1 tablespoon maple syrup

Grease two ramekins with the butter and set aside.

Heat the dates and water in a small saucepan over a low heat until the dates break down and thicken. Set to one side.

Place the coconut flour, egg, banana, vanilla bean paste and baking powder in a blender or food processor and mix until well combined and aerated.

Gently combine the date and banana mixtures and evenly distribute into the ramekins. Cook in a microwave oven at 80 per cent power for 2.5 minutes or until springy in the middle.

While the puddings are in the microwave, place the sticky date syrup ingredients in a small saucepan over a low heat and cook for about 2 minutes or until the dates start to break down but are still slightly chunky.

Allow the puddings to rest for a minute before turning them out onto serving plates, then pour over the sticky date syrup and serve.

Oh my, this pudding is so decadent and sweet! To be enjoyed occasionally, but when you do—enjoy it thoroughly!

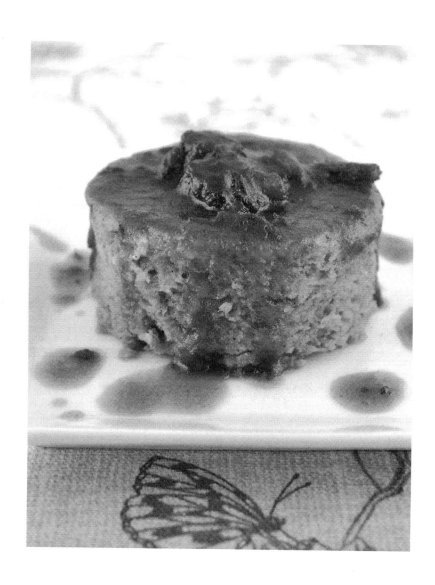

Ingredients Glossary

ACTIVATED NUTS AND SEEDS: To activate your nuts and seeds, cover them in water and soak them for around 12 hours or overnight. Drain and rinse well, then dehydrate them. If using a dehydrator, dehydrate them according to the dehydrator's instructions. If using an oven, spread out the nuts and seeds on baking trays lined with baking paper and bake at your oven's lowest temperature (70–100°C/150-200°F) with the door slightly ajar, until crisp. Activate all of your nuts and seeds before using them. The soaking helps remove some of the anti-nutrients found in the seeds and nuts, such as phytic acid, and the dehydrating at a low temperature reduces damage to the good oils found in the nuts and seeds. After activating your nuts and seeds, store them in an airtight container in the fridge. This also helps to protect the oils, preventing them from going rancid.

ASIAN SHALLOTS: Originating in Central or Southwest Asia, Asian shallots belong to the same genus as the onion *(Allium)* but have a milder flavour. They are generally reddish in colour and are often interchanged with red onions.

CACAO BUTTER: Derived from the natural fat extracted from cacao beans during the process of making cacao powder, cacao butter is a rich source of anti-oxidants and is mainly used to make chocolate, although it can be used as a skin moisturiser. It is found in all good health-food stores.

CACAO NIBS: These are simply raw cacao beans crushed up to a crumbly texture. They contain omega-3s, zinc and have amazing levels of magnesium. They are great for adding texture and a chocolaty crunch to desserts and drinks. They are found in good health-food stores.

CACAO POWDER: The raw form of cocoa powder, raw cacao powder has not been processed at high temperatures like cocoa powder and therefore retains all of its nutritional qualities. It is found in all good health-food stores.

CHIA SEEDS: *Salvia hispanica* or chia is a member of the mint family and is native to central and southern Mexico and Guatemala. The seeds from this plant are a rich source of omega-3 fatty acids as well as calcium and manganese. Chia seeds are commonly used as a topping in foods such as smoothies and yoghurt or to make puddings.

CHINESE FIVE-SPICE: An aromatic mix of five ground spices (star anise, Szechuan pepper, fennel seeds, cinnamon and cloves) commonly used in Chinese cooking.

COCONUT AMINOS: This is the highly nutritious sap produced by tapping coconut trees. It's raw, low glycaemic and has an abundance of amino acids and other minerals and vitamins. Less salty than tamari sauce (See section entitled "Ingredients Glossary") it's a great substitute for soy sauce, which is a definite no-no. It is found in specialty health-food stores.

COCONUT SUGAR: Coconut sugar is produced from the sap of cut flowerbuds of the coconut palm and has been used as a natural sweetener in South-East Asian cuisine for thousands of years. Rich in potassium, magnesium, zinc and iron, it has a subtle sweet flavour with a slight hint of caramel. It is found in good health-food stores or can be purchased online.

DULSE: Often referred to as 'sea lettuce', dulse is an edible red seaweed commonly found on the northern coasts of the Atlantic and Pacific oceans. Mainly sold as flakes, dulse has the highest iron content of any food and its briny, pungent flavour is used in soups and condiments.

FLAX SEEDS: Also known as linseeds, flax seeds are the seeds of the flax plant and can be used whole or ground to make flax meal. They are rich in B vitamins and antioxidants. They can be found in most supermarkets.

GHEE: Ghee is clarified butter, which means the milk proteins have been removed and what is left is just the butter fat. It can generally be used interchangeably with butter. You can find ghee in most supermarkets, health-food stores or Asian grocers.

HORSERADISH: Fresh horseradish is the root of the horseradish plant. It is very pungent and hot, but adds a wonderful kick to dishes. Store-bought horseradish is not as hot as the fresh stuff. You can generally find fresh horseradish at farmers' markets.

KELP NOODLES: Made from the sea vegetable kelp, kelp noodles are gluten free and low in carbohydrates. They are made purely from kelp, sodium salt extracted from brown seaweed and water. They are a great alternative to gluten-containing noodles, but tend to lend themselves more to Asian-inspired dishes. They can be found in health-food stores or purchased online.

MARINATED ARTICHOKE: Artichoke hearts marinated in a mixture of olive oil, vinegar and herbs and spices can be found in most supermarkets. Just be aware that commercially manufactured marinated artichokes are sometimes marinated using seed oils such as canola or safflower oil, which you want to avoid where possible.

MEDJOOL DATES: Originating from the Middle East and North Africa, dates are the fruit of date palms. Medjool dates are known for their large size, sweetness and juicy flesh even when dried, and make a great Paleo sweetener. You can find them in most supermarkets in the fruit and vegetable section.

NORI: *Nori* is the Japanese name for edible seaweed. Originally from Japan, nori sheets are made by turning nori into dried, paper-thin, black square sheets about 20cm (8in) in size. You can find these in most large supermarkets or at your local Asian grocer.

NUTRITIONAL YEAST: Nutritional yeast should not be confused with Brewer's yeast. Nutritional yeast is a dried inactive yeast from the *Saccharomyces cerevisiae* strain. It is packed with B vitamins and adds a lovely nutty, cheesy flavour. Sold as flakes in a container or packet, nutritional yeast can be found in good health-food stores.

PANDANUS LEAVES: Pandanus leaves come from Pandanus palms and are used a lot in Asian cooking for both sweet and savoury dishes. You can find them at most Asian grocers.

PINK HIMALAYAN SALT: Pink Himalayan salt contains a full spectrum of trace minerals such as magnesium, calcium, iodine and iron and is still in its natural, unrefined form. It is available from good supermarkets and health-food stores.

RAW HONEY: This is the natural, unheated, unpasteurised and unprocessed honey obtained straight from extraction. There may by some pollen and other particles in the honey giving it a cloudy appearance. The absence of the heating process preserves all of the nutrients and enzymes. Raw honey should be avoided by pregnant women and young children and babies. It is available from good health-food stores.

ROSEWATER: During the process of making rose oil, rose petals and water are distilled and the leftover liquid is rosewater. It has a distinctive rose smell and florally taste, which can be quite strong. It is commonly used in Middle Eastern cooking. You can find it in most supermarkets or specialty cooking stores.

SAMBAL: A chilli-based condiment used in Asian cooking, sambal may also contain other ingredients such as garlic, ginger and lemongrass. It is found in some supermarkets or Asian grocers.

SAWTOOTH CORIANDER: Also called long or wild coriander, sawtooth coriander has long leaves with serrated edges, hence the name 'sawtooth'. It is used extensively in Vietnamese cooking and is similar to common coriander, but with a much stronger flavour. It is found in specialty Asian grocers.

SUMAC: A powder ground from the fruits of shrubs from the genus Rhus. Grown throughout the Middle East and the Mediterranean, the spice is used to add a tangy lemony flavour and is one of the main spices that makes up a za'atar mix. It is available from most supermarkets or specialty food stores.

TAMARI SAUCE: Although soy sauce and tamari are both made from fermented soybeans, Japanese tamari is thicker, darker and richer. It has a more complex, smoother flavour than soy sauce and comes in gluten-free versions. It is available from supermarkets and Asian grocers.

TRUFFLE OIL: This oil is used to give the subtle hint of truffles to a dish. Truffles are the fruiting body of fungi that grow under the ground. They are highly prized and have a very strong, pungent, earthy taste and smell. It is available at specialty food stores or online.

TURMERIC: The rhizome (underground stem) of the turmeric plant, this spice can be used fresh or ground as a dried powder. It has a slightly bitter, mustardy flavour with a lovely rich orangey/yellow colour and contains curcumin, a powerful anti-inflammatory. Ground turmeric can be found in most supermarkets and fresh turmeric at Asian grocers or farmers markets.

VANILLA BEAN PASTE: The inside of vanilla bean pods, scraped out into a small jar. It is available from specialty food stores.

Conversion Tables

OVEN TEMPERATURES

°CELSIUS (C)	°FAHRENHEIT (F)
120	250
150	300
180	355
200	400
220	450

WEIGHT EQUIVALENTS

METRIC	IMPERIAL (APPROXMATE)
10g	1/3oz
50g	2oz
80g	3oz
100g	3 1/2oz
150g	5oz
175g	6oz
250g	9oz
375g	13oz
400g	14oz
500g	1lb
750g	1 2/3lb
1kg	2lb

VOLUME EQUIVALENTS

METRIC	IMPERIAL (APPROXMATE)
20ml	1/2fl oz
60ml	2fl oz

METRIC	IMPERIAL (APPROXMATE)
80ml	3fl oz
125ml	4 1/2fl oz
160ml	5 1/2fl oz
180ml	6fl oz
250ml	9fl oz
375ml	13fl oz
500ml	18fl oz
750ml	1 1/2 pints
1 litre	1 3/4 pints

CUP AND SPOON CONVERSIONS

1 teaspoon	5ml
1 tablespoon	20ml
1/4 cup	60ml
1/3 cup	80ml
1/2 cup	125ml
2/3 cup	160ml
3/4 cup	180ml
1 cup	250ml

Acknowledgements

It truly has been an amazing experience writing this book, and there is no way I could have done it without the huge amount of support from so many. I really do have many people to thank!

Paul, Abi and Betty Yates—my gorgeous family. Thank you, my amazing husband and best friend. There is just no way I could have done this without you. You have been my chief photographer, editor, computer-tech support and just about EVERYTHING! Your support never wavers and you have helped me every step of the way. You had the confidence in me when I didn't and you have allowed me to shine—thank you! I love you and I love adventuring through life with you. My two little 'fur babies' Abi and Betty—thank you for your wet kisses and 'stress therapy'. You guys are magical and just light up my life.

Mum and Dad—thank you for always believing in me and telling me, even from a young age, that I could do anything I put my heart into. I love you guys.

Janine Flanagan—my sister, chief editor and cheer squad. You helped me so much when you were SO busy with your own work and always gave me the pep talk I needed. I thank you from the bottom of my heart and I love you.

429

Liv Butcher—thank you for always being there when I needed you and for sending over emergency supplies. ☺ You kept Paul and me going.

Wendy Brissenden—my amazing naturopath! Thank you for keeping me alive with supportive herbs and equally supportive chats.

Irena Macri—thank you for sharing one of your prized recipes with me. I look forward to more amazing creations from you in the future.

Lola Berry—thank you for your continual sound advice and support, and for sharing your recipe in this book.

Beth McGregor—thank you for your feedback and your technical eye! I really appreciate it.

Warren Maginn—thank you for your time, knowledge and technical expertise. I really appreciate all you have contributed to this book.

Anouska, Monica, Tracey and the Exisle team—thank you for giving me this opportunity and for having such patience with me! You have been amazing.

References

Chapter 1

World Health Organization's definition of health: http://www.who.int/about/definition/en/print.html

Chapter 2

Albarracin W, Sanchez IC et al. (2011). Salt in food processing; usage and reduction: a review. *International Journal of Food Science & Technology,* 46(7): 1329–36.

Alvheim AR, Malde MK et al. (2012). Dietary linoleic acid elevates endogenous 2-AG and anandamide and induces obesity. *Obesity* (Silver Spring), 20(10): 1984–94.

Ameur A, Enroth S et al. (2012). Genetic adaptation of fatty-acid metabolism: a human-specific haplotype increasing the biosynthesis of long-chain omega-3 and omega-6 fatty acids. *American Journal of Human Genetics,* 90(5): 809–20.

Bateman B, Warner JO et al. (2004). The effects of a double blind, placebo controlled, artificial food colourings and benzoate preservative challenge on hyperactivity in a general population sample of preschool children. *Archives of Disease in Childhood,* 89(6): 506–11.

Baumgart K. (2012). Allergic rhinitis. *Medical Observer,*http://www.medicalobserver.com.au/news/allergic-rhinitis

Berzas Nevado JJ et al. (1998). Resolution of ternary mixtures of Tartrazine, Sunset yellow and Ponceau 4R by derivative spectrophotometric ratio spectrum-zero crossing method in commercial foods. *Talanta,* 46(5): 933–42.

Cederroth CR, Auger J et al. (2010). Soy, phyto-oestrogens and male reproductive function: a review. *International Journal of Andrology,* 33(2): 304–16.

Dowdee A and Ossege J. (2007). Assessment of childhood allergy for the primary care practitioner. *Journal of the American Academy of Nurse Practitioners,* 19(2): 53–62.

Eady J. (2006). *Additive Alert: Your guide to safer shopping,* Additive Alert Pty Ltd, Mullaloo, WA.

Kashanian S and Zeidali SH. (2011). DNA binding studies of tartrazine food additive. *DNA and Cell Biology,* 30(7): 499–505.

L'Hocine L and Boye JI. (2007). Allergenicity of soybean: new developments in identification of allergenic proteins, cross-reactivities and hypoallergenization technologies. *Critical Reviews in Food Science and Nutrition,* 47(2): 127–43.

Nordic Naturals. (2013). How do we know we are deficient?. Nordic Naturals website, retrieved 23/2/2013: http://www.nordicnaturals.com/training/pdfs/TheBigFatStory_22513.pdf

Norrman G, Tomicic S et al. (2005). Significant improvement of eczema with skin care and food elimination in small children. *Acta Paediatrica,* 94(10): 1384–8.

Osiecki H. (2008). *The Nutrient Bible* 7th ed., Bio Concepts Publishing, Eagle Farm, QLD.

Prescott S and Allen KJ. (2011). Food allergy: riding the second wave of the allergy epidemic. *Pediatric Allergy and Immunology,* 22(2): 155–60.

Prescott SL, and Tang ML. (2005). The Australasian Society of Clinical Immunology and Allergy position statement: Summary of allergy prevention in children. *Medical Journal of Australia,* 182(9): 464–7.

Ramsden CE, Ringel A et al. (2012). Lowering dietary linoleic acid reduces bioactive oxidized linoleic acid metabolites in humans. *Prostaglandins, Leukotrienes and Essential Fatty Acids,* 87(4–5): 135–41.

Simopoulos AP. (2006). Evolutionary aspects of diet, the omega-6/omega-3 ratio and genetic variation: nutritional implications for chronic diseases. *Biomedicine & Pharmacotherapy,* 60(9): 502–7.

Theobald HE. (2005). Dietary calcium and health. *British Nutrition Foundation Nutrition Bulletin,* 30(3): 237–77.

Voruganti VS, Higgins PB et al. (2012). Variants in CPT1A, FADS1 and FADS2 are associated with higher levels of estimated plasma and Erythrocyte Delta-5 Desaturases in Alaskan Eskimos. *Frontiers in Genetics,* 3:86.

Chapter 3

Allison AJ and Clarke AJ. (2006). Letter to the editor: Further research for consideration in 'the A2 milk case'. *European Journal of Clinical Nutrition,* 60: 921–4.

A2 Dairy Products Australia Pty Ltd. Beta-casein, retrieved 01/04/2013: http://www.betacasein.org/

Biesiekierski JR, Newnham ED et al. (2011). Gluten causes gastrointestinal symptoms in subjects without celiac disease: a double-blind randomized placebo-controlled trial. *American Journal of Gastroenterology,* 106(3): 508–14.

434

Cederroth CR, Auger J et al. (2010). Soy, phyto-oestrogens and male reproductive function: a review. *International Journal of Andrology,* 33(2): 304–16.

Choi J, Sabikhi L et al. (2012). Bioactive peptides in dairy products. *International Journal of Dairy Technology,* 65(1): 1–12.

De Punder K, and Pruimboom L. (2013). The dietary intake of wheat and other cereal grains and their role in inflammation. *Nutrients,* 5(3): 771–87.

Gaudin JC, Rabesona H et al. (2008). Assessment of the immunoglobulin E-mediated immune response to milk-specific proteins in allergic patients using microarrays. *Clinical & Experimental Allergy,* 38(4): 686–93.

Hill JP, Crawford RA and Boland MJ. (2002). Milk and consumer health: a review of the evidence for a relationship between the consumption of beta-casein A1 with heart disease and insulin-dependent diabetes mellitus. *Proceedings of the New Zealand Society of Animal Production,* 62, 111–4.

Jaminet P and Jaminet SC. (2013). *Perfect Health Diet,* Scribe Publications, Brunswick, Victoria.

Lestienne I, Mouquet-Rivier C et al. (2005). The effects of soaking of whole, dehulled and ground millet and soybean seeds on phytate degradation and Phy/Fe and Phy/Zn molar ratios. *International Journal of Food Science & Technology,* 40(4): 391–9.

Macdonald K and Macdonald TM. (2010). The peptide that binds: a systematic review of oxytocin and its prosocial effects in humans. *Harvard Review of Psychiatry,* 18(1): 1–21.

Nachbar MS and Oppenheim JD. (1980). Lectins in the United States diet: a survey of lectins in commonly consumed foods and a review of the literature. *American Journal of Clinical Nutrition,* 33(11): 2338–45.

Ramadass B, Dokladny K et al. (2010). Sucrose co-administration reduces the toxic effect of lectin on gut permeability and intestinal bacterial colonization. *Digestive Diseases and Sciences,* 55(10): 2778–84.

Sanwalka JN, Khadilkar AV et al. (2011). Development of non-dairy, calcium-rich vegetarian food products to improve calcium intake in vegetarian youth. *Current Science,* 101: 657–63.

Sapone A, Bai JC et al. (2012). Spectrum of gluten-related disorders: consensus on new nomenclature and classification. *BMC Medicine.* 10:13.

Seiquer I, Delgado-Andrade C et al. (2010). Assessing the effects of severe heat treatment of milk on calcium bioavailability: in vitro and in vivo studies. *Journal of Dairy Science,* 93(12): 5635–43.

Teschemacher H, Umbach M et. al. (1986). No evidence for the presence of beta-casomorphins in human plasma after ingestion of cows' milk or milk products. *Journal of Dairy Research,* 53(1), 135–8.

Theobald HE. (2005). Dietary calcium and health. *British Nutrition Foundation Nutrition Bulletin,* 30(3): 237–77.

Truswell AS, (2005). The A2 milk case: a critical review. *European Journal of Clinical Nutrition,* 59(5): 623–31.

Truswell AS. (2006). Reply: The A2 milk case: a critical review. *European Journal of Clinical Nutrition,* 60(7), 924–5.

Venkata Raman B, Sravani B et al. (2012). Effect of plant lectins on human blood group antigens with special focus on plant foods and juices. *International Journal of Research in Ayurveda & Pharmacy,* 3(2): 255.

Woodford KB. (2006). A critique of Truswell's A2 milk review. *European Journal of Clinical Nutrition,* 60(3), 437–9.

Yoshikawa M, Takahashi M et al. (2003). Delta opioid peptides derived from plant proteins. *Current Pharmaceutical Design,* 9(16): 1325–30.

Chapter 4

Bagger JI, Knop FK et al. (2011). Glucagon antagonism as a potential therapeutic target in type 2 diabetes. *Diabetes, Obesity and Metabolism,* 13(11): 965–971.

Cardona Cano S, Merkestein M et al. (2012). Role of ghrelin in the pathophysiology of eating disorders: implications for pharmacotherapy. *CNS Drugs,* 26(4): 281–96.

Edwards LD, Heyman AH et al. (2011). Hypocortisolism: an evidence-based review. *Integrative Medicine,* 10(4): 26–33.

Hou N and Luo J. (2011). Leptin and cardiovascular diseases. *Clinical and Experimental Pharmacology and Physiology,* 38(12): 905–13.

Klimas NG and Koneru AO. (2007). Chronic fatigue syndrome: inflammation, immune function, and neuroendocrine interactions. *Current Rheumatology Reports,* 9(6): 482–87.

Lindmark S, Buren J et al. (2006). Insulin resistance, endocrine function and adipokines in type 2 diabetes

438

patients at different glycaemic levels: potential impact for glucotoxicity in vivo. *Clinical Endocrinology,* 65(3): 301–9.

Pranjic N, Nuhbegovic S et al. (2012). Is adrenal exhaustion synonym of syndrome burnout at workplace? *Collegium Antropologicum.* 36(3): 911–9.

Roper J, Francois F et al. (2008). Leptin and ghrelin in relation to Helicobacter pylori status in adult males. *Journal of Clinical Endocrinology & Metabolism,* 93(6): 2350–7.

Schmid SM, Hallschmid M et al. (2008). A single night of sleep deprivation increases ghrelin levels and feelings of hunger in normal-weight healthy men. *Journal of Sleep Research,* 17(3): 331–4.

Scott MM, Williams KW et al. (2011). Leptin receptor expression in hindbrain Glp-1 neurons regulates food intake and energy balance in mice. *Journal of Clinical Investigation,* 121(6): 2413–21.

Skibicka KP, Hansson C et al. (2012). Role of ghrelin in food reward: impact of ghrelin on sucrose self-administration and mesolimbic dopamine and acetylcholine receptor gene expression. *Addiction Biology,* 17(1): 95–107.

Taheri S, Lin L et al. (2004). Short sleep duration is associated with reduced leptin, elevated ghrelin, and increased body mass index. *PLOS Medicine,* 1(3): e62.

Taneja SK, Mandal R et al. (2012). Attenuation of Zn-induced hyperleptinemia/leptin resistance in Wistar rat after feeding modified poultry egg. *Nutrition & Metabolism,* 9(1): 85.

Chapter 5

Baldwin et al. (2003–4). Playing games for self-esteem. *McGill Reporter,* 36, McGill University, Canada.

Edwards LD, Heyman AH et al. (2011). Hypocortisolism: an evidence-based review. *Integrative Medicine,* 10(4): 26–33.

Hébert, S, Béland R et al. (2005). Physiological stress response to video-game playing: the contribution of built-in music. *Life Sciences,* 76: 2371–80.

Klimas NG and Koneru AO. (2007). Chronic fatigue syndrome: inflammation, immune function, and neuroendocrine interactions. *Current Rheumatology Reports,* 9(6): 482–87.

Pranjic N, Nuhbegovic S et al. (2012). Is adrenal exhaustion synonym of syndrome burnout at workplace? *Collegium Antropologicum.* 36(3): 911–9.

Chapter 6

Cerf-Bensussan N and Gaboriau-Routhiau V. (2010). The immune system and the gut microbiota: friends or foes? *Nature Reviews Immunology,* 10(10): 735–44.

De Palma G, Nadal I et al. (2010). Intestinal dysbiosis and reduced immunoglobulin-coated bacteria associated with coeliac disease in children. *BMC Microbiology,* 10:63.

Hawrelak JA and Myers SP. (2004). The causes of intestinal dysbiosis: a review. *Alternative Medicine Review.* 9(2): 180–97.

Koplin J, Allen K et al. (2008). Is caesarean delivery associated with sensitization to food allergens and IgE-mediated food allergy: a systematic review. *Pediatric Allergy & Immunology,* 19(8): 682–7.

Lutgendorff F, Akkermans LM et al. (2008). The role of microbiota and probiotics in stress-induced gastro-intestinal damage. *Current Molecular Medicine,* 8(4): 282–98.

Moreno-Navarrete JM, Sabater M et al. (2012). Circulating zonulin, a marker of intestinal permeability, is increased in association with obesity-associated insulin resistance. *PLoS One.* 7(5): e37160.

Osiecki, H. (2008). *The Physician's Handbook of Clinical Nutrition,* Bio Concepts Publishing, Eagle Farm, QLD.

Wood S, Pithadia R et al. (2013). Chronic alcohol exposure renders epithelial cells vulnerable to bacterial infection. *PLoS One* 8(1): e54646.

Chapter 7

Elks CM and Francis J. (2010). Central adiposity, systematic inflammation, and the metabolic syndrome. *Current Hypertension Reports,* 12(2): 99–104.

Hannestad J, Subramanyam K et al. (2012). Glucose metabolism in the insula and cingulate is affected by systemic inflammation in humans. *Journal of Nuclear Medicine,* 53(4): 601–7.

Krysiak R, Gdula-Dymek A et al. (2011). The effect of bezafibrate and omega-3 fatty acids on lymphocyte cytokine release and systemic inflammation in patients with isolated hypertriglyceridemia. *European Journal of Clinical Pharmacology,* 67(11): 1109–17.

Richette P, Poitou C et al. (2011). Benefits of massive weight loss on symptoms, systemic inflammation and cartilage turnover in obese patients with knee osteoarthritis. *Annals of Rheumatic Diseases,* 70(1): 139–44.

Chapter 8

Pears P. (2006). *Organic Gardening in Australia.* Dorling Kindersley Australasia, Camberwell, Victoria.

Pitchford P. (2002). *Healing with Whole Foods: Asian traditions and modern nutrition.* North Atlantic Books, Berkeley, California.

Chapter 9

Jaminet P and Jaminet SC. (2013). *Perfect Health Diet,* Scribe Publications, Brunswick, Victoria.

Osiecki, H. (2008). *The Physician's Handbook of Clinical Nutrition,* Bio Concepts Publishing, Eagle Farm, QLD.

Chapter 10

Cho YY, Kwon EY et al. (2011). Differential effect of corn oil-based low trans structured fat on the plasma and hepatic lipid profile in an atherogenic mouse model: comparison to hydrogenated trans fat. *Lipids in Health and Disease,* 10:15.

D'Archivio M, Filesi C et al. (2010). Bioavailability of the polyphenols: status and controversies. *International Journal of Molecular Science,* 11(4): 1321–42.

Gillingham LG, Harris-Janz S et al. (2011). Dietary monounsaturated fatty acids are protective against metabolic syndrome and cardiovascular disease risk factors. *Lipids,* 46(3): 209–28.

Gómez-Alonso S, Fregapane G et al. (2003). Changes in phenolic composition and antioxidant activity of virgin olive oil during frying. *Journal of Agricultural and Food Chemistry,* 51(3): 667–72.

Greenberg JA, Bell SJ et al. (2008). Omega-3 fatty acid supplementation during pregnancy. *Reviews in Obstetrics & Gynecology,* 1(4): 162–9.

Harman NL, Leeds AR et al. (2008). Increased dietary cholesterol does not increase plasma low density lipoprotein when accompanied by an energy-restricted diet and weight loss. *European Journal of Nutrition,* 47(6): 287–93.

Hu FB, Manson JE et al. (2001). Types of dietary fat and risk of coronary heart disease: a critical review. *Journal of the American College of Nutrition,* 20(1): 5–19.

Liau KM, Lee YY et al. (2011). An open-label pilot study to assess the efficacy and safety of virgin coconut oil in reducing visceral adiposity. *ISRN Pharmacology,* 2011:949686.

444

Mahan KL and Escott-Stump S. (2008). *Krause's Food and Nutrition Therapy* 12th ed., Saunders Elsevier, St Louis, Missouri.

Nakatsuji T, Kao MC et al. (2009). Antimicrobial property of lauric acid against Propionibacterium acnes: its therapeutic potential for inflammatory *acne vulgaris. Journal of Investigative Dermatology,* 129(10): 2480–8.

Nasser R, Cook S et al. (2011). Consumer perceptions of trans fats in 2009 show awareness of negative effects but limited concern regarding use in snack foods. *Applied Physiology, Nutrition & Metabolism,* 36(4): 526–32.

Nettleton JA, Lutsey PL et al. (2009). Diet soda intake and risk of incident metabolic syndrome and type 2 diabetes in the Multi-Ethnic Study of Atherosclerosis (MESA). *Diabetes Care,* 32(4): 688–94.

[No authors listed]. (1984). The Lipid Research Clinics Coronary Primary Prevention Trial results. I. Reduction in incidence of coronary heart disease. *Journal of the American Medical Association,* 251(3): 351–64.

Sartorius T, Ketterer C et al. (2012). Monounsaturated fatty acids prevent the aversive effects of obesity on locomotion, brain activity, and sleep behavior. *Diabetes,* 61(7): 1669–79.

SELF Nutrition Data. 'Nutritional Information: Fish & Chips', retrieved 2/2/2013: http://nutritiondata.self.com/facts/recipe/2771712/2

SELF Nutrition Data. 'Nutritional Information: Grilled Fish', retrieved 2/2/2013: http://nutritiondata.self.com/facts/recipe/2771669/2

Siri-Tarino PW, Sun Q et al. (2010). Meta-analysis of prospective cohort studies evaluating the association of saturated fat with cardiovascular disease. *American Journal of Clinical Nutrition,* 91(3): 535–46.

Statin Nation. (2013). Statin Nation Fact Sheet 1, Statin Nation website, retrieved 14/3/2013: http://www.statinnation.net/storage/STATIN_NATION_FactSheet1.pdf

Chapter 11

Bjelakovic G, Nikolova D et al. (2012). Antioxidant supplements for prevention of mortality in healthy participants and patients with various diseases. *Cochrane Database of Systematic Reviews,* 3:CD007176.

Braun L and Cohen M. (2007). *Herbs & Natural Supplements: An evidence-based guide.* Elsevier Australia, Marrickville, New South Wales.

Choudhary N and Sekhon BS. (2012). Potential therapeutic effect of curcumin—an update. *Journal of Pharmaceutical Education & Research,* 3(2): 64–9.

Eliassen AH, Missmer SA et al. (2008). Circulating 2-hydroxy- and 16-alpha-hydroxy estrone levels and risk of breast cancer among postmenopausal women. *Cancer Epidemiology, Biomarkers & Prevention,* 17(8): 2029–35.

Food Standards Australia New Zealand. (2011). Mercury in Fish, Food Standards Australia New Zealand website, retrieved 16/4/2013: http://www.foodstandards.gov.au/consumerinformation/mercuryinfish.cfm

Jin Y. (2011). 3,3'-Diindolylmethane inhibits breast cancer cell growth via miR-21-mediated Cdc25A degradation. *Molecular & Cellular Biochemistry,* 358(1–2): 345–54.

Minich DM and Bland JS. (2007). A review of the clinical efficacy and safety of cruciferous vegetable phytochemicals. *Nutrition Reviews,* 65(6 Pt 1): 259–67.

Orthoplex. EstroClear Technical Information. Orthoplex, 2011. http://www.bioconcepts.com.au

Pears P. (2006). *Organic Gardening in Australia.* Dorling Kindersley Australasia, Camberwell, Victoria.

Pitchford P. (2002). *Healing with Whole Foods: Asian traditions and modern nutrition.* North Atlantic Books, Berkeley, California.

Rathee P, Chaudhary H et al. (2009). Mechanism of action of flavonoids as anti-inflammatory agents: a review. *Inflammation & Allergy—Drug Targets,* 8(3): 229–35.

Moncayo R, Kroiss A et al. (2008). The role of selenium, vitamin C, and zinc in benign thyroid diseases and of selenium in malignant thyroid diseases: Low selenium levels are found in subacute and silent thyroiditis and in papillary and follicular carcinoma. *BMC Endocrine Disorders,* 8:2.

SELF Nutrition Data. 'Nutritional Facts and Analysis: Fish, salmon, Atlantic, wild, raw', retrieved 23/2/2013: http://nutritiondata.self.com/facts/finfish-and-shellfish products/4102/2

Triggiani V, Tafaro E et al. (2009). Role of iodine, selenium and other micronutrients in thyroid function and disorders. *Endocrine, Metabolic & Immune Disorders—Drug Targets,* 9(3): 277–94.

Tripathi S, Bruch D et al. (2008). Ginger extract inhibits LPS induced macrophage activation and function. *BMC Complementary & Alternative Medicine,* 8: 1.

Vattem DA, Lester CE et al. (2012). Dietary supplementation with two *Zingiberaceae* spices ginger and turmeric modulates innate immunity parameters in *Lumbricus terrestris. Journal of Natural Pharmaceuticals,* 3(1): 37–45.

Xu J, Yang XF et al. (2006). Selenium supplement alleviated the toxic effects of excessive iodine in mice. *Biological Trace Element Research,* 111(1–3): 229–38.

Chapter 12

Aloulou A, Hamden K et al. (2012). Hypoglycemic and antilipidemic properties of kombucha tea in alloxan-induced diabetic rats. *BMC Complementary & Alternative Medicine,* 12:63.

Anderson RC, Cookson AL et al. (2010). Lactobacillus plantarum DSM 2648 is a potential probiotic that enhances intestinal barrier function. *FEMS Microbiology Letters,* 309(2): 184– 92.

Bajpai M, Mishra A et al. (2005). Antioxidant and free radical scavenging activities of some leafy vegetables. *International Journal of Food Sciences & Nutrition,* 56(7): 473–81.

Barrett JS, Irving PM et al. (2009). Comparison of the prevalence of fructose and lactose malabsorption across chronic intestinal disorders. *Alimentary Pharmacology & Therapeutics,* 30(2): 165–74.

Chen YP, Hsiao PJ et al. (2012). Lactobacillus kefiranofaciens M1 isolated from milk kefir grains ameliorates experimental colitis in vitro and in vivo. *Journal of Dairy Science,* 95(1): 63–74.

Davidson LE, Fiorino AM et al. (2011). Lactobacillus GG as an immune adjuvant for live-attenuated influenza vaccine in healthy adults: a randomized double-blind placebo-controlled trial. *European Journal of Clinical Nutrition,* 65(4): 501–7.

Department of Health and Ageing, National Health and Medical Research Council, Australian Government. (2006). Nutrient reference values for Australia and New Zealand: including recommended dietary intakes. NHMRC: http://www.nhmrc.gov.au/_files_nhmrc/publi cations/attachments/n35.pdf

Eutamene H and Bueno L. (2007). Role of probiotics in correcting abnormalities of colonic flora induced by stress. *Gut,* 56(11): 1495–7.

Hendricks JM, Hoffman C et al. (2012). 18β-glycyrrhetinic acid delivered orally induces isolated lymphoid follicle maturation at the intestinal mucosa and attenuates rotavirus shedding. *PLoS One,* 7(11): e49491.

Isaacs J. (2009). *Bush Food: Aboriginal food and herbal medicine.* New Holland Publishers (Australia), Chatswood, New South Wales.

Khan J and Islam MN. (2011). Intestinal barrier function: impairment and possible modulation. *International Medical Journal,* 18(3): 212.

Li Q, Zhang Q et al. (2011). Fish oil enhances recovery of intestinal microbiota and epithelial integrity in chronic rejection of intestinal transplant. *PLoS ONE,* 6(6): e20460.

Miettinen M, Pietilä TE et al. (2012). Nonpathogenic Lactobacillus rhamnosus activates the inflammasome and antiviral responses in human macrophages. *Gut Microbes,* 3(6): 510–22.

Morcos A, Dinan T et al. (2009). Irritable bowel syndrome: role of food in pathogenesis and management. *Journal of Digestive Disorders,* 10(4): 237–46.

Sedin F. (2010). Ancient Kombucha. *Alive: Canada's Natural Health & Wellness Magazine,* 329:40.

Siebecker A and Sandberg-Lewis S. (2013). Small intestine bacterial overgrowth: often-ignored cause of irritable bowel syndrome. *Townsend Letter,* 355/356:85.

Versalovic J, Iyer C et al. (2008). Commensal-derived probiotics as anti-inflammatory agents. *Microbial Ecology in Health and Disease,* 20(2): 86–93.

Yapar K, Cavusoglu K et al. (2010). Protective effect of kombucha mushroom (KM) tea on phenol-induced cytotoxicity in albino mice. *Journal of Environmental Biology,* 31(5): 615–21.

Zakostelska Z, Kverka M et al. (2011). Lysate of probiotic Lactobacillus casei DN-114 001 ameliorates colitis by strengthening the gut barrier function and changing the gut microenvironment. *PLoS One,* 6(11): e27961.

Chapter 13

Anderson RC, Cookson AL et al. (2010). Lactobacillus plantarum MB452 enhances the function of the intestinal barrier by increasing the expression levels of genes involved in tight junction formation. *BMC Microbiology,* 10:316.

Braun L and Cohen M. (2007). *Herbs & Natural Supplements: An evidence-based guide.* Elsevier Australia, Marrickville, New South Wales.

Gigante G, Tortora A et al. (2011). Role of gut microbiota in food tolerance and allergies. *Digestive Diseases,* 29(6): 540–9.

Nermes M, Kantele JM et al. (2011). Interaction of orally administered Lactobacillus rhamnosus GG with skin and gut microbiota and humoral immunity in infants with atopic dermatitis. *Clinical & Experimental Allergy*, 41(3): 370–7.

Pärtty A, Kalliomäki M et al. (2012). Compositional development of Bifidobacterium and Lactobacillus microbiota is linked with crying and fussing in early infancy. *PLoS ONE* 7(3): e32495.

Chapter 14

Aksungar FB, Topkaya AE et al. (2007). Interleukin-6, C-reactive protein and biochemical parameters during prolonged intermittent fasting. *Annals of Nutrition & Metabolism.* 51(1): 88–95.

Feinman RD. (2011). Fad diets in the treatment of diabetes. *Current Diabetes Reports,* 11(2): 128–35.

Heilbronn LK, Civitarese AE et al. (2005). Glucose tolerance and skeletal muscle gene expression in response to alternate day fasting. *Obesity Research.* 13(3): 574–81.

Heilbronn LK, Smith SR et al. (2005). Alternate-day fasting in nonobese subjects: effects on body weight, body composition, and energy metabolism. *American Journal of Clinical Nutrition.* 81(1): 69–73.

Kumar S and Kaur G. (2013). Intermittent fasting dietary restriction regimen negatively influences reproduction in young rats: a study of hypothalamo-hypophysial-gonadal axis. *PLoS ONE,* 8(1): e52416.

Michalsen A. (2010). Prolonged fasting as a method of mood enhancement in chronic pain syndromes: a review of clinical evidence and mechanisms. *Current Pain & Headache Reports.* 14(2): 80–7.

Novotny JA, Gebauer SK et al. (2012). Discrepancy between the Atwater factor predicted and empirically measured energy values of almonds in human diets. *American Journal of Clinical Nutrition,* 96(2): 296–301.

Tomiyama A, Moskovich A et al. (2009). Consumption after a diet violation: disinhibition or compensation? *Psychological Science,* 20(10): 1275–81.

Varady KA, Bhutani S et al. (2009). Short-term modified alternate-day fasting: a novel dietary strategy for weight loss and cardioprotection in obese adults. *American Journal of Clinical Nutrition,* 90(5): 1138–43.

Varady KA and Hellerstein MK. (2007). Alternate-day fasting and chronic disease prevention: a review of human and animal trials. *American Journal of Clinical Nutrition.* 86(1): 7–13.

Chapter 15

Hackney AC, Kallman A et al. (2012). Thyroid hormonal responses to intensive interval versus steady-state endurance exercise sessions. *Hormones,* 11(1): 54–60.

Liu Y, Croft JB et al. (2013). Association between perceived insufficient sleep, frequent mental distress, obesity and chronic diseases among US adults, 2009 behavioral risk factor surveillance system. *BMC Public Health,* 13:84.

Morselli LL, Guyon A et al. (2012). Sleep and metabolic function. *Pflugers Archive,* 463(1): 139–60.

Schmid SM, Hallschmid M et al. (2008). A single night of sleep deprivation increases ghrelin levels and feelings of hunger in normal-weight healthy men. *Journal of Sleep Research,* 17(3): 331–4.

Taheri S, Lin L, Austin D et al. (2004). Short sleep duration is associated with reduced leptin, elevated ghrelin, and increased body mass index. *PLoS Med,* 1(3): e62.

Wells ME and Vaughn BV. (2012). Poor sleep challenging the health of a nation. *Neurodiagnostic Journal,* 52(3): 233–49.

Chapter 19

Osiecki H. (2008). *The Nutrient Bible* 7th ed., Bio Concepts Publishing, Eagle Farm, Queensland.

Osiecki, H. (2008). *The Physician's Handbook of Clinical Nutrition,* Bio Concepts Publishing, Eagle Farm, Queensland.

Chapter 20

Osiecki H. (2008). *The Nutrient Bible* 7th ed., Bio Concepts Publishing, Eagle Farm, Queensland.

Osiecki, H. (2008). *The Physician's Handbook of Clinical Nutrition,* Bio Concepts Publishing, Eagle Farm, Queensland.

Chapter 21

Osiecki H. (2008). *The Nutrient Bible* 7th ed., Bio Concepts Publishing, Eagle Farm, Queensland.

Osiecki, H. (2008). *The Physician's Handbook of Clinical Nutrition,* Bio Concepts Publishing, Eagle Farm, Queensland.

Back Cover Material

Eating the Paleo way is not about becoming a 'caveman'! Instead, it's all about listening to your body, getting back to a more natural, seasonal way of eating, **nourishing your body** with tasty whole foods and living a more balanced lifestyle. Along the way, you'll automatically **consume far less sugar,** avoid preservatives and processed foods, and **throw away the calorie counter for good!**

In *Optimum Health the Paleo Way,* Paleo nutritionist Claire Yates explains clearly why bad health is on the increase and how the Paleo lifestyle (not 'diet') can help. Along the way, you'll also **discover the truth about fats, carbs, protein and fibre,** and how you can **use 'food as medicine'** to improve and then maintain your health.

By following the 28-day Reset protocol, you'll be able to design **an individual Paleo food plan** that works for you, and with over 100 delicious recipes to try you'll soon be feeling great while eating some of the tastiest food of your life!